To Vicki

ASCENT OF A WOMAN

Mhairi Blyth

Thank you

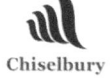
Chiselbury

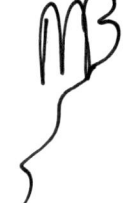

Published by Chiselbury Publishing, a division of Woodstock Leasor Limited, 14 Devonia Road, London N1 8JH, United Kingdom

www.chiselbury.com

The moral right of Mhairi Blyth to be identified as the author of this work is asserted.

This work is copyright material and must not be copied, reproduced, transferred, distributed, leased, licensed or publicly performed or used in any way except as specifically permitted by the publishers, as allowed under the terms and conditions under which it was purchased or as strictly permitted by applicable copyright law. Any unauthorised distribution or use of this text may be a direct infringement of the publisher's rights and those responsible may be liable in law accordingly.

Chiselbury Publishing hereby exclude all liability to the extent permitted by law for any errors or omissions in this book and for any loss, damage or expense (whether direct or indirect) suffered by any third party relying on any information contained in this book.

ISBN: 978-1-916556-65-2 (hardback)

ISBN: 978-1-908291-66-9 (epub)

Cover design by Indra Murugiah

© Mhairi Blyth 2025

To all those in their ascent…

TABLE OF CONTENTS

Prologue 1
Chapter 1 5
Chapter 2 13
Chapter 3 19
Chapter 4 29
Chapter 5 37
Chapter 6 49
Chapter 7 60
Chapter 8 66
Chapter 9 72
Chapter 10 78
Chapter 11 84
Chapter 12 96
Chapter 13 106
Chapter 14 117
Chapter 15 126
Chapter 16 134
Chapter 17 142
Chapter 18 148
Chapter 19 155
Chapter 20 164
Chapter 21 173
Chapter 22 178
Chapter 23 190
Chapter 24 197
Chapter 25 205
Chapter 26 212
Acknowledgements 217

PROLOGUE

By now I was all too familiar with the metal taste developing in my mouth. The blood spotting in my pants had started an hour or so earlier though I had tried to ignore it. It wasn't unusual for me to get blood spotting with having Endometriosis, but I knew the difference by now. An almighty pain tore through my womb, unlike anything I had ever felt before, even with my seven other babies. But this baby was older. Bigger. At nearly ten weeks, my baby had managed to hold on longer than any other. I had begun to secretly hope and believe that my dream was finally coming true. How foolish was I to think everything would be fine this time. The pain was so intense it made me throw up. It was like a knife ripping though my womb. Raw and stabbing. And then the bleeding really started. Heavy and unrelenting, most of the day until, after dinner, as I was sitting on the toilet, unsure if I was going to be sick or have the runs, I felt what I thought was a massive blood clot fall away from me and plop into the toilet. I got up, turned round, and peered into the toilet bowl.

   I shouldn't have. My baby was lying lifeless at the bottom. I knew it wasn't just a blood clot because I could clearly see the shape of a baby in miniature, its little head, limbs, and dark spots for eyes. Nothing in this world can prepare you for that. That was it for me. I cracked. I didn't care about the blood running down my legs and the mess on the floor. I just sat against the bath, crying, cradling my baby I'd so carefully scooped up out of the bottom of the toilet bowl. Some people say there is no 'human baby' at this point in a pregnancy, but let me tell you, when you are sitting staring closely, tracing every outline, memorising every feature, when you can see that what you are holding in your bloody, shaking hand, when you can see that what your own body has rejected is a baby, in your mind there is no other form it could take. When you see that, when you really look at it, you never forget it. That image of your baby stays with you. Every. Single. Day.

I don't know how much time passed, but eventually I realised I was now sitting in a cold, congealing pool of blood and needed to clean myself up. Why, I don't know, but I wrapped my baby in toilet roll before putting it back in the toilet and saying goodbye. Then I got started, cleaning first myself, then the bathroom floor. I phoned Simon, but there was no answer.

"Simon," I cried down the phone. "Please can you come home early? It's happened again. I've lost the baby, Simon. I'm so sorry. I don't know what to do. Hopefully you get this."

He didn't come home early.

When he did get home from working his night shift the next morning, there was no talking about it. I kept apologising for days, but his response was always the same. It's okay, it's not your fault. But that was as far as it went. There was no holding each other and sharing in the loss, letting the tears flow onto each other's shoulders and consoling each other. Just my frequent apologies and his one-line reply.

In the September, when the pain was beginning to sting a little less, I was again reminded of my body's repeated failed attempts to give me a baby naturally. I was offered an appointment in Aberdeen for IVF treatment, which I knew all too well I wouldn't be able to handle. Simon replied, telling them what had happened, and politely declining the offer.

***

After the miscarriage, and the lack of support from Simon, I began to regret buying the house together. He worked shifts and regularly took overtime, often only letting me know while on the shift already, or just before he went in, that he wouldn't be home on time, or at all that night. I threw myself into work at the bookies as well and was back and forth to Inverness to help Mum with Dad whenever I could get across to them. Most of the time, Mum would drive half an hour to come and get me but that meant bringing Dad too. Sometimes he wasn't able to come out of the house and he couldn't be left himself in the house anymore.

Simon and I were like ships in the night, and barely saw each other. We'd recently got a little puppy, a blue roan cocker spaniel whom I named Breagha, the Gaelic for beautiful; and she was, and still is. She became my little baby, following me everywhere I went and cuddling up to me on the sofa against my hot water bottle when I was in pain. We were inseparable.

Only a month after we declined the invitation for IVF, Simon told me one of his work colleagues was expecting. "What do you think to maybe giving IVF a shot after all?" he asked me one night.

I was shocked. We'd just refused the offer from the Aberdeen clinic. I wasn't in a fit state yet to start thinking of that. In fact, I didn't think I ever would be fit to think about it. Years of pain, and loss and mental anguish. That was the last straw for me. I didn't want my periods, didn't want endometriosis, didn't want IVF, didn't want to be told what to do with my body, didn't want to be told that unfortunately there wasn't much else that could be done as it was just 'one of those things', or 'just part of being a woman'. I was sick of being told I was 'too young to make that sort of decision'. I was done with it all.

"No way!" I told him. "I can't do it again. I can't put my body or my mind through that pain again. I'm done trying for a baby. I'm done being told I'm too young to decide about my own body myself. I'm done being everybody else's puppet."

He glared at me. It wasn't a sympathetic stare, nor a questioning look of I'm not sure I understand. It was a glare, pure and simple.

"You are kidding," he said.

"No, I am not kidding, Simon. I am done. Completely done."

"What about me?"

"I'm sorry, what? What about you? It's my body. My decision. And I'm done."

"Surely you can try those pills again."

That was it for me. That was the moment I switched off. He hadn't hit me. He'd been annoyed, but he hadn't shouted at me. He hadn't come at me or threatened me. But that moment, standing in the kitchen, was just as bad in my eyes as a smack in the face. It was just as bad as Nick and Michael. In that moment, my body, my feelings, and my whole being were about to be claimed for something I didn't consent to. I was tired of doctors telling me what to do with my body. I was tired of being pushed in directions I didn't want to go. My whole life had been a series of where other people and events had decided what way my life would go. But losing my eighth baby was my breaking point. It was time to take back some control of my life.

CHAPTER 1

I came into this world like a baseball flying into my dad's ungloved hands on February 1, 1984. So eager was I to make an appearance that there was barely any time for the midwives to gown up and ready the labour suite. Luckily, Dad was a nurse and knew what he was doing, so I was quite safe, and soon was being cooed over at home by my proud parents, Allan and Joyce Hutt.

My first house was in Lower Largo, Fife, Scotland, the home of Alexander Selkirk, whose buccaneering, castaway life inspired Daniel Defoe's Robinson Crusoe. There's even a wee statue of him in the village. Life was uneventful and normal for the first two years of my existence – Dad worked a lot as a nurse in Victoria Hospital, Kirkcaldy, and Mum looked after me and my two half-sisters, Sharon, and Lesley. Money was scarce, but with some careful budgeting and counting slices of bread, we all ate, had clothes, and were housed. Interest rates under Thatcher's government went through the roof, meaning unaffordable increases to our mortgage, so Dad took an opportunity to work abroad as a nurse in Jeddah, Saudi Arabia, taking us with him. So in 1986, we emigrated.

Of course, being two at the time, I've no memory of this at all. My first memory is of being in our apartment in Jeddah, listening to Queen's 'It's a Kind of Magic' and 'One Vision', while Mum did housework. Then there are other silly little memories like the Humpty Dumpty cake Mum made me for my third birthday, with half-melted icing, or watching sandstorm clouds roll in across the desert landscape from the living room window, then having gritty eyes because of the dusty residue that had sneaked into the flat through the air conditioner units. The residue caused havoc on the marble floors, making them painful to walk on in bare feet, which was how I almost always walked around the house. Even worse than sand on a marble floor was any type of liquid. One morning Lesley, who was nine at the time, was making us both breakfast. She put the bread in the toaster, and we waited.

"Aah!" she screamed, running out of the room. "Dad! Dad! Fire!" It was then that I noticed the orange flickers coming from the toaster. I ran out of the kitchen into the hall to see Lesley standing at the other end of the living room, outside Mum and Dad's bedroom, her face bright red and sniffling. I heard some frustrated-sounding muffles for a few seconds before Dad came flying into the room, completely nude, swearing as he slid on little streaks of pee that Lesley had left in her wake on the way through to the kitchen. How he managed to stay upright and get the fire blanket over the toaster I'll never know, but he was my superhero that day.

It was in Jeddah that I was introduced to swimming for the first time. The grounds of our apartment complex had a large swimming pool with loungers where families gathered to socialise, and I became a little water baby. I took to the water very easily and I didn't really use armbands or floats. Instead, I swam freely, both underwater and at the surface, with just my big black-and-yellow goggles to protect my eyes. I loved swimming as far as I could underwater before coming up for a quick breath and going back under again. For me, it was the calm under the water that felt so good. With my whole body supported by the water, I would kick my wee legs to propel myself along the pool. I spent hours and hours in the pool, and it quickly became my favourite place to be. The whole two years in Jeddah were lovely. We were all together as a family, a normal family, and the memories that I can recall were happy and funny and pure and innocent. I was innocent.

***

We returned to Fife in 1989 when I was five. We stayed in Kirkcaldy, where I went to the local primary school and made wee pals, as you do. Sharon and Lesley were nine and six years older than me respectively, so they had their own lives at school and their own pals. To some extent I was an only child. We never really had that sisterly bond and, as is often the case with siblings, they didn't want me round them bugging them every two minutes. Instead I depended on Mum and Dad quite heavily, possibly more than was necessary, to compensate for a lack of relationship with my sisters. That's why, when Dad was offered another contract in Saudi Arabia, and accepted, my little world broke a little. This time he would be going alone, with the promise that we could join him as soon as things could be organised. I was devastated. My dad was leaving us; leaving me. It was very confusing, trying to understand that nothing bad was happening, even though my dad was going to live somewhere else. It felt like the family was breaking up, and I didn't know when I'd see Dad again.

The first Gulf War was brewing, and I remember listening to Mum and Dad sometimes talking about the dangers when they thought I was asleep. I often heard flashes of the news from the television and they'd constantly flash through my brain as I tried to make sense of the situation. Dad was going to Al Khobar on the east coast, just over 200 miles from the Kuwait border. He would be in a compound for expats and the area had air bases and troops from the UK and America nearby. I gathered we wouldn't be following any time soon, because he was going to a dangerous place. When Dad left, I was six, and I didn't know if I would ever see him again.

"Are you behaving, Mhairi? Please don't act up for your mum," he would say to me over the phone.

"I miss you! Please come home, Dad!" I used to cry back. My behaviour changed after Dad left. I would stay up incredibly late, creeping about the house, seeing how much I could get up to without getting caught. In my bedroom, there was a sloped wall which had a Velux window, decorated with a piece of material held up by white plastic-covered wire with loops at the end, pulled over hooks in the wood to make a curtain. Opposite this, I had a wee open wardrobe with white-panelled walls, and at the back was a small door which opened into the attic space. It was like The Lion, The Witch and The Wardrobe, my own little Narnia, and I used to sit in there for ages with the door slightly ajar, cuddling my big white teddy, Snowflake. I'd got him from Mum and Dad the Christmas before Dad went away, and I'd sit and talk to him, in the place where nobody could see me.

"Are you okay, Dad? I miss you." I'd wait patiently for the reply. "Please come home, Dad. I love you." Snowflake remained silent but I liked to think that Dad could hear me anyway.

My other favourite place to hide was the back of my cabin bed. It was completely white, with drawers down the middle and a cupboard at each end. The actual bed sat above the drawers and cupboards. I loved that bed for two reasons. Firstly, it was huge, like my very own castle, with walls round the mattress that you had to scale just to go to sleep, and you'd have to jump down to the floor when you wanted to get out. Secondly, both cupboards had these flimsy backboards held on by three nails each, that bent whenever anything pressed against them. In all my wisdom I had knocked those backboards off to create a cave under my castle where I could hide from everyone. If I couldn't sleep, I just used to hide in the attic space or in my cave under the bed with Snowflake, and somehow it calmed me down.

The downside of all my night-time shenanigans was how tired I was during the day. I wasn't getting enough sleep to help me concentrate at school, or anywhere for that matter. I even missed out on my cameo role as the nativity donkey because I fell asleep in the classroom reading corner. The less I slept, the more tired I became, and the more tired I became, the more irritated I became, which led to me becoming angry and grumpy. My concentration span became almost non-existent, and nothing ever seemed to be enough to occupy me. What made things worse was that the first Gulf War was by now in full flow, and phone calls from Dad became less about his recollections of what he'd been up to recently, and more about him trying to stay safe in a war zone.

"I heard this almighty whistle, louder than anything I've heard before," he said. "And then not a minute later a huge explosion lit up the night sky." That was the night a missile hit an ammunition dump a few miles away from the compound.

Other times he'd tell me about his work. "Today it was quiet in the clinic, but we kept ourselves busy by taping up all the windows. We had to tape all around the edges of the glass, then tape big crosses in the middle in case the windows get blown in by blasts from exploding missiles. Then our new uniforms came. We've each got a full camouflage suit and a gas mask. I look ridiculous in it. We've taken photos. I'll send them in my next letter." He'd chuckle whilst he told me, like he was making light of the situation. But my night-time excursions to halfway down the stairs led me to piece together the reality of the dangerous situation that Dad was in, and I remember thinking we would never be reunited. I'd sit and listen to Mum talking to Dad on the phone. If she was talking a lot and laughing, I knew he was okay, and that was all I needed to know. It was when she went quiet that I got nervous.

"Mm ... Mm ... what was that? Missile?" I heard the tremors in her voice many times, and I was scared too. I'd sit on the olive-green nylon carpet on the stairs and stare at the wall, trying not to cry out.

***

We lived in a Victorian semi-detached house just outside Kirkcaldy town centre. Our street was a mile long, from the hospital at the top to the promenade at the bottom, and was filled with working families and couples. The ceilings in the house were high and had massive plaster ceiling roses surrounding all the light fittings and decorative plaster coving round the edges to match. The walls were made of horsehair plaster and though the house was generally in good condition, it needed a tidy up here and there. There wasn't much to be doing when I was sat on the stairs at night, and I would trace the lumps and bumps on the wall to keep me occupied whilst earwigging. I didn't realise that this old plaster was brittle so when I found a little hole with a few hairs sticking through, naturally I pulled at them. Then I pulled at the ones that appeared next, and the ones after that, and before I knew it there were a few holes in the wall. Not just little pinholes that are easy to hide, but proper chunks of plaster and horsehair had come off the wall, assisted by my little busy fingers.

"Just you wait till I get home!!" Dad would yell down the phone. "You'll get a hot arse for that!"

True to his word, when he came home, I'd get the promised punishment. My trousers and pants would come down, and he'd stick me over his knee and skelp me. I could often see my sisters half giggling, half wincing, as I ran upstairs screaming to my cave under the bed. In my mind all I wanted was for my dad to come home but then, when he did, I got smacked. Having Dad so far away was awful, but when he first came home for holidays, it was horrible too. He was always back for at least two weeks so by the time he went away again, the smacks had been forgotten, my behaviour had improved, and I was back to square one, not wanting him to go away and wondering why he had to.

Another time, I gave Mum's dressing table stool a makeover. She had one of those 'fashionable' bedroom furniture suites, with wall-to-wall shiny, mahogany veneer, from the three-drawer bedside cabinets to the double pedestal dressing table, with a tri-folding mirror, and a lovely, pink velvet cushioned stool to match. I locked myself in her bedroom one day to hide from her threats of phoning Dad for my misbehaving. At first, she didn't know where I was, and after a short while I got bored, so I started rummaging through the dressing table drawers. I found some pink and red nail polishes, and took them out. Then I started to paint the stool with them. Nothing artistic, just blobs here and stripes there. I thought it looked lovely to be honest, an original masterpiece.

"Mhairi! Where are you? Come here right now!"

I stayed quiet.

"Mhairi?"

I heard footsteps coming up the stairs.

"Are you in here?"

She was in my room. Then the door handle rattled.

"Mhairi? Are you in there? What are you doing in there? You better not be doing anything naughty."

I looked at the stool. Uh oh! I need to get this off quick.

"Coming, Mum."

I looked in the drawer and pulled out the nail polish remover and started dribbling it all over my artwork.

"Let me in now!" Mum yelled. Realising the nail polish remover wasn't just removing the polish, but also the plush coating of the stool, I knew the game was up. I unlocked the door and let Mum in.

"What have you done? Wait till your dad hears about this!"

"I'm sorry," I snivelled. "Don't tell Dad. I'm sorry, Mum!"

"It's too late now. He'll be so disappointed to hear you've been naughty again!"

It was just another thing to add to the 'naughty list' for Dad to deal with when he got home. Top tip ... do not use nail polish remover on pink velvet, it takes the surface off the material super quick and leaves a sort of flattened appearance that's rough to the touch.

It didn't matter to me if I was good or bad, Dad was still away. We came back from Jeddah when I was five, and for the next three years I was constantly seen as the naughty one, when all I really wanted was for us to be a family again.

CHAPTER 2

I calmed down early in 1992, when I was eight and it became clear we were to be reunited with Dad. The Gulf War was over, and it was finally safe to go to Saudi Arabia. Houses were made available for families like ours. Lesley was fourteen and in high school, and Sharon was seventeen. They both had established friendship groups and didn't want to come, so they stayed with Nana and Papa in Kirkcaldy. To me, this was the best news ever. Mum and I would be going to live with Dad in Saudi. Getting off the plane at Dhahran International Airport was like walking into an oven; everything was baked brown. Light brown, dark brown, beige. Even the greenery had hues of being roasted brown at some point. There was a light breeze, but it was midsummer so the blast of hot hair that hit me was overwhelming. Nevertheless, the recently war-torn land felt familiar and, ironically, safe.

We went to our new house, which was on a complex with three family compounds and three bachelor sections. As we greeted the security guard and went through the barriers to our new compound, I was surprised to see separate bungalows, all lined up neatly rather than the high-rise apartment blocks that had littered the Jeddah countryside back in 1986. Every bungalow had little front gardens with the odd palm tree and aloe vera plant scattered around. I could see gardeners hard at work, sweeping paths and pruning the bougainvillea bushes that lined the compound walls. Ours was a small bungalow towards the rear of the compound. Nothing extravagant, but just enough for the three of us.

I loved spending time outside. The roads were smooth with the occasional speed bump, perfect for riding my shiny new red bike everywhere and anywhere within the compound's walls. There was a bowling alley, table tennis rooms and a shop where I used to spend my pocket money on American treats: Hershey's Kisses, Nerds and Lay's crisps. There were two playparks I spent hours in. One was small with a swing set and a metal slide that burnt your legs on the way down, having soaked up the forty-degree summer sun. There were parallel bars that I would swing around and hang upside-down from, before crashing onto the hot sand below. The other playpark was much bigger and featured a massive dome of metal bars in the middle that looked like one of those spun sugar domes you get on posh desserts. The crowning glory for me though had to be the choice of three swimming pools. I had barely done any swimming in the three years since Jeddah, so I was looking forward to making the most of them.

Then there was school, Dhahran Academy. To make allowances for the heat, it started at eight in the morning and finished around two. The ride there was about half an hour in a big white bus, like the yellow school buses you see in America. Mum was a monitor on the buses and had to check the bus for bombs every morning. Cars were checked on entry to the compounds too – a legacy of the recent war. The school hadn't escaped the war either and I remember being frightened for the first few weeks that I went there.

Dhahran Academy had the misfortune (or fortune, depending how you look at it) of sitting next to an American airbase. The sprawling car park of the school was patrolled by Saudi guards, riding armoured vehicles with mounted guns. There were two guards on each truck: a driver and a guard manning the gun, scanning the grounds for threats. There were armed guards with bayonets on the gates to the school and every person going in got scanned with metal detectors before being allowed to walk up the hill to the main campus.

We got introduced to air raid drills the first week, rather than just fire drills too. The sirens would start screeching and if we were in a classroom we had to get under the nearest desk as quickly as possible. If you were milling about outside, you'd hear frantic squeals and shouts as we ran to the nearest wall to crouch behind or toilet block to get under a sink. It was a far cry from forming an orderly line and walking to the nearest assembly point back in Kirkcaldy. The first few times it was scary, and I remember on more than one occasion seeing other kids crying and having to be comforted by the teachers. It was all too real when we heard the thundering of a military plane down the runway next door and then the roar of the engine overhead as it passed the school. Thankfully nothing ever happened for real, but the drills never stopped, and the guards were always present in the car park, waiting just in case.

When I wasn't at school, Mum and I went on days out to the local shops where I would buy the latest Kylie Minogue cassette, or a pair of earrings from one of the many jewellers. My favourite shop was Al Zamil's, which was a massive craft shop over two floors. I loved buying cross-stitch threads and kits, treating myself to pencils and notepads, or kitting myself out with new folders to organise stuff in. I noticed that all the women, from mid-teens upwards, including Mum, would walk around covered head to toe in their black abayas, some with only their eyes visible. All the kids my age dressed in normal kids' clothes.

"Why do you need to wear that, Mum?"

"When we go out, we must cover up like everybody else. We need to make sure we abide by the rules. You don't need to do that until you're a bit older though."

I was grateful, because the abayas looked so restrictive, and adding layers in the desert heat wasn't appealing. I remember one day being out with Mum. We saw two women outside the compounds without an abaya. They were being approached by local men and women shouting at them in Arabic.

"What's happening, Mum?" I asked her.

"Just stay close to me, okay. That's the Mutawa. They're religious police. They're angry at those women for not covering up."

"What about those Saudi women?"

"You watch, they'll start surrounding them in a minute. They don't like foreigners disrespecting their rules. Women need to be seen and not heard here. If they find out who their husbands are, they will get in trouble from their employers. Some even get sent home." Sure enough, as we stood watching from across the street, the Saudi women started surrounding the two women. They ushered them into a nearby shop and Mum and I continued walking. "They'll keep them there until they either get some form of abaya on or their husbands pick them up."

"When will I need to get an abaya? I don't want to get Dad into trouble."

"Not for a while yet. Don't worry, we will take you to get one when it's time."

When the three of us weren't at school or work, we'd travel an hour or so to the beach that the expat communities used. It was a massive stretch of shoreline that had been walled off for our use, with men, women and children allowed to wear regular swimwear without fear of reprimand. We could all use the local beaches, but no swimwear was allowed unless you were a child. They were less for sunbathing than walking along. I remember Dad's initial lecture about staying safe in the sun. The Saudi heat was fierce, and you could burn very quickly with the worst cases needing hospitalisation for heat stroke and first-degree burns. Some people would be in for days at a time on drips to rehydrate them again.

"You need to wear sunscreen all the time, Mhairi. Head to toe and absolutely no baby oil. I've seen people in the clinic with burns because they've used baby oil." Dad was stood in front of me while I was sat on the white plastic patio chair waiting to go to the beach. He was smoking a cigarette and had his car keys at the ready.

"Yes, Dad."

"Please stay in the shade between 11am and 3pm, because that's when it is hottest in the day. You might get heatstroke if you don't, okay?" He was checking I was listening properly. He'd often do that, ask me a question when he'd told me something just to make sure it had stuck in my head.

"Okay, I'll stay in the shade, I promise. Can we go now?"

He turned towards the gate as if ready to finally go but then turned back and pointed the car keys at me. "And you must drink lots of fluids. If you don't, you'll get ill. You can get very ill and even die." He nodded and walked out the gate, satisfied he'd covered everything.

"Aye, okay Dad, I hear you."

He was right with his advice, of course, and I did follow it, until one day a few months later when we were at the beach I saw him slap baby oil on himself in the morning when we got there and then he lay out in the baking heat all day in his yellow budgie smugglers, listening to his Walkman.

"What happened to 'no baby oil'?" I asked.

"I'm used to it," he grinned from under his cream bucket hat. How he didn't end up in his own clinic, I don't know.

I'd spend most of my time in the sea. I'd only come out of the water to eat or drink, then go straight back in again. Mum would flit between chatting to the other mums and soaking up the sun with Dad, and would only occasionally come in the shallow area, as she feared the deeper water.

Sometimes, when it got too hot for even Dad to lie there baking, he'd shout for me to come back.

"Get the snorkels and masks, Mhairi. Let's go and feed the fish." He'd rummage around in his bag for an empty water bottle with some bread in it. I'd run up to our loungers and get the snorkels and masks out of my beach bag before turning round and running towards the sea again.

"Yeah, come on then! Race you!" I'd yell back, whilst getting a head start.

There was a big yellow American school bus which had been sunk on purpose just past the sand ledge where the shallow water gave way to deeper water. I'd swim down to the bus with Dad, with my snorkel and mask on, and squeeze the bottle which had the bits of bread in it to fill it with water, then squeeze it again to let some mushy bread out. Loads of little shimmering fish would hurriedly swim up to the bread cloud, then open their little mouths to get a feed.

These were fun days, and those first couple of years from August 1992 were by far the happiest part of my childhood. I naively thought my life would always be like those two years, when everything felt easy. I even loved getting woken up with a start at five o'clock in the morning by the local Imam calling out for morning prayers from the mosque. His voice was always so boomingly loud and crisp. It was, without a doubt, an order to get up and get to the mosque. It always started so suddenly that I would wake up with a jolt, wondering what was happening, then sink back into my pillow and listen to his morning song. It became familiar and comforting. A sign, to me, that I was where I loved being and that Mum, Dad and I were together.

CHAPTER 3

It was November 1993 and I'd been in Saudi with Mum and Dad for little over a year. I was so happy that when Mum and Dad sat me down in the living room after tea one night to talk to me about something important, I could never imagine what was about to happen.

"Your mum and I have been looking at schools for you. It's time you went back to Scotland as you're getting to high school age and the education will be far better back home." Dad had his reading glasses on and he was peering over them. It was his serious look. From the moment they told me I would need to go back to Scotland to school, and that I'd be living at the school, my life as I knew it ended.

"But all my friends are here. Nobody in my year is going anywhere yet. I've got another year before I'm high school age," I protested.

"Yes, but you won't get the same standards here. It's for the best, Mhairi," Mum replied. "We are thinking of your future."

"I don't think you are. I'm happy here. I want to stay with you. Don't you want me here? Can I not just stay an extra year and then I'll go?"

"No, Mhairi. It's time just now. We just want what's best for you," Mum said.

"No, you just want rid of me!" I started to raise my voice and I could feel the tears burning in my eyes. "You're sending me thousands of miles away because you don't want me here any more. At least be honest about that!"

"It's for your own good, Mhairi," Dad quipped back rather loudly. "It's all organised! Your nana and papa and sisters will only be half an hour away and you'll see them at weekends and half-term. You can come back here at the end of each term and in the summer."

"It's not for my own good at all. Lesley and Sharon won't visit me. They don't care about me," I cried as I got off the seat and went towards my room. "You just want rid of me," I yelled and slammed my bedroom door behind me. There was no point in arguing any more. The decision had been made for me already and I was going to boarding school in Edinburgh whether I agreed to it or not. I still refused to believe I was going until I got dropped off at the school in August 1994.

"We'll see you in a few weeks, Mhairi. Keep your chin up and work hard," Dad said. "It will go quick, you'll see."

"I'll write to you when we get back home and see how you're doing, okay?" Mum added.

"Please, please don't leave me here. I can't do this. It's horrible," I begged.

"Now give it a chance. I'm sure you'll have lots of fun and make friends," Dad replied. Mum and Dad left me there, sobbing on the bed. It seemed all too easy for them to leave me without either of them shedding a tear. That was it – I was ten years old and alone, feeling abandoned by my parents, in a place full of strangers who didn't know the first thing about me and who didn't care about me. The person I was before August 1994 vanished.

***

The all-girls school was made up of three boarding houses which were Victorian built. Each had a large, heavy front door which led into a cold, tiled hallway with the housemistress's office on the right, a large common room to the left and a smaller sitting room a little up the hallway.

Farther still was a small kitchen and a laundry room with a wooden door to the left which led to the canteen and school grounds. On the right, the stone staircase had a thick, black, metal banister, which doubled back on itself up towards the second floor. Here were three dorms, a communal bathroom and a small staircase leading up to the housemistress's rooms. Everything just looked functional and nothing like home. It felt as though I was walking through a scene from a bad dream. The floors were cold, the banister was cold, the woodwork was cold. The place had no heart.

My dorm would be the first on the right; a massive room with walls painted off-white, bay windows on two sides and colossally high ceilings. Half of the room had a rough cream-coloured floor, and the other half had thin, worn, dark blue carpet tiles. There were five beds, but only four of us in the room, each with a grey, metal bed frame, with a thin mattress, a wonky bedside cupboard, and a badly built single wardrobe. None of the furniture was matching, instead the room looked like it had been furnished from car boot sales. There was a single, yellowing duvet, and one flat pillow on each bed. I felt sick that I would have to live here. It was like something out of the orphanage on Annie.

Unsurprisingly, we were all homesick, and all we had was each other so we formed close bonds, quite quickly getting to know where each other was from and who our families were.

"My parents are in Germany," said Flora. "They're in the army so this is probably the longest I'll have ever been in one place. Does anyone like running? I sometimes go running with my mum before breakfast."

"Absolutely not," said Diane. "Back in Qatar the sea's so warm, I could lie in it all day. What about you, Lorraine?"

"My parents are in Hong Kong. No running or swimming for me. I go shopping with my mum a lot. Or out to lunch with her friends. I'll miss that."

"My parents are in Saudi Arabia, but my sisters and grandparents are in Fife, just across the Forth bridge. I'm hoping I can see them most weekends," I said. "They're just half an hour away."

Initially, it wasn't a bad place to be. We were just a bunch of ten-year-olds trying to get along in a very strange place, and we became friends. We would sit together chatting and giggling at mealtimes in the canteen and, whilst we did our compulsory homework time at nights, we'd pass each other silly notes, trying not to get caught by whoever was monitoring the session that night, because if you got caught, you'd have to sit by yourself the next night.

We had little outings at the weekend, when we would go down to the local high street, and even wear our own clothes. We always went to the sweet shop first to buy giant gobstoppers with our couple of pounds of pocket money, even though there were old, half-eaten ones back in the dorms. It didn't matter what we bought, really; it was a small weekly taste of normality for those that were still there at the weekend. Lots of the girls went to relatives at the weekend, some travelling up to two hours to come and collect them. It was nearing the October break of 1994 and my nana; papa and two sisters hadn't managed to come and see me yet. I'd received letters from them, and from my parents in Saudi.

When Nana and Papa came to pick me up for the October half-term week I was absolutely delighted, as it had been two months since I'd had any real contact with any of my family. My sisters had moved out to a house five minutes away from Nana and Papa, which Mum and Dad provided for them, so I got a bedroom all to myself, which I treasured so much, having had to share a room with four others at school. I was so grateful to be in a familiar setting for a while, and I felt even better knowing I would speak to my parents in Saudi that week.

"Yes, I've been behaving ... I'm having lots of fun ... making friends, yes ... miss you ... love you ... can't wait to come home at Christmas." I was being genuine when I said it; I was having fun and making friends and behaving. For all my protestations about being sent away, it had so far turned out to be nowhere near as bad as I imagined it would be.

When I got taken back to school, there were a couple of new girls who had arrived in the house. One was just eight, so she went into in the younger girls' room across the hall. Then there was a girl who came into our dorm, who was two years older. There wasn't any room in any other dorms, so she was given the empty bed beside us. She didn't say too much about herself, and we didn't see a lot of her during the daytime, as she hung around with the girls her own age. After a couple of weeks went by, I started noticing a shift in our group; three of the girls started hanging about together more, chatting amongst themselves, almost distancing themselves from the rest of the dorm. The youngest girl in our dorm started to spend more time in another dorm, and by default the older girl and me were left with each other. She was in a situation like me, in that she never really went away at weekends, so there were a few incidents when we were left alone, and that's when it started.

One weekend we were sat talking after lights out, and she asked if I wanted to play a game: sandbags. Curious, I agreed, as I'd never heard of this game from the other girls.

"Okay," she said, "First you need to lie on your back and spread your arms and legs out like a starfish. So, I'm going to make it feel like I'm cutting your arms and legs open and then I'm going to fill them up with sand and then stitch them back up again, so you feel heavy and stuck to the bed. It'll make you feel tired and then it'll be easy for you to go to sleep." So, as instructed, I lay flat on my back like a starfish. She started pretending to slice down each arm slowly and carefully with her fingernails.

"It tickles!" I laughed out loudly.

"Just shut your eyes. Eventually it won't tickle. It'll just feel comforting."

I shut my eyes and tried to stop my giggles by concentrating on the motion of her fingers on my arms. Then she kneaded the sand into my arms, packing it in tightly, filling them up to the brim. Then the criss-cross action of closing my arms back up having rendered them immobile. I wriggled a little.

"No, don't move them, they're full of sand, remember?" she reminded me. "Okay, legs now. Stay there."

I felt the same scratchy sensation of slits being made on my legs with her fingernails, followed by the deep pressure of her kneading the sand into my legs before criss-crossing the openings shut, securing my sand-laden legs in one place. I giggled again.

"That was fun. Thanks. I need to get up, though." I started to move and went to get up off the bed.

"No, you can't move yet, they're full of sand so stay there because I'm going to do your tummy now." It was like a friendly order, so I didn't say anything back, just nodded my head whilst she stood over me and unbuttoned my pyjama shirt.

"What are you doing?" I asked.

"Your tummy. Stop moving!" Again, I felt her fingernails slicing from my neck to the waistband of my pyjama bottoms, kneading the sand into my stomach then criss-crossing the sand into place. I laughed again and went to get up when she pushed me back down.

"I really need to move. It tickles a lot and I need the toilet. Thanks, though."

"Well, you have to stay lying down because you're full of sand so stay there."

There was an anger to her voice I'd never heard before and it shocked me, so I just lay back down, only this time there was no getting up voluntarily, because she came up on the bed and knelt on my thighs. What happened next seemed to be all part of the game to her, as she performed the 'sandbags' routine over my bare torso. She thought it was funny, giggling as she carried it out. I just lay there in disbelief with tears rolling down my temples and onto the bed. When she was finished, she just got off me and went to her bed without a word. I lay there for a few moments then pulled the covers over me and lay in the foetal position whilst crying myself to sleep.

In the morning, it was as though nothing had happened, and when other boarders started returning later that day, the events of the night before seemed to have been forgotten about. Everything went back to normal for a while, until a couple of weeks later, when we were the only two left at the weekend again.

"Let's play sandbags."

"No, I'm okay. I'm quite tired."

"Well, I want to play it." And she got out of bed and came over to mine.

This time there wasn't any giggling, and by the time it was over, I was lying completely naked, sprawled out on my bed. I avoided her the next day, instead I stuck to places where we wouldn't be alone. When the others came back, I was so relieved because it meant I didn't have to be alone with her at night. And when the holidays came, I practically ran down the stairs to greet my nana and papa. I didn't want to go back to school this time, and I cried a lot when I got dropped back at the front door.

A few days after we were all back, Cheryl introduced 'sandbags' to the dorm one night, as a game she thought would be fun for us all to play. She showed everyone how to play using my arms and said it was made better if you sat on each other because it felt as though you were heavy. So, everyone joined in, picked their partners, and played along. This time she skipped the legs and went straight on with my chest and groin. After she'd finished, I remember her leaning down, grabbing a chunk of my hair, and pulling very hard whilst she told me to keep quiet. It was the same angry tone I'd heard before and I was petrified. I just did what she said. Most nights the dorm would play whilst she pretended to play along and every night, I'd end up crying myself to sleep. My moods started to change as I became too tired to concentrate on schoolwork and I started to kick back against the rigid routines and strict rules of boarding school life. When the others were away, I did my best to stay away from the dorm and when they were back, I'd stick to them like glue. I became angry and resentful at being left behind at the weekend when my family were only half an hour away. The housemistress had me in her office on many occasions: she knew something was wrong, but I never told her anything, other than that I wanted to go home, and I hated being there.

***

I can't remember Mum coming to get me from the school, but I do recall we went to stay with my sisters for a week or so while we waited to go back to Saudi. I'd been taken out of school for reasons unknown to me and Mum had to fly from Saudi back to Edinburgh to get me.

"I'm taking you to Kirkcaldy, to stay with Lesley and Sharon for a while until we organise a flight back to Saudi," Mum had shouted at me. "God knows what you've done or what's happened, but you are not going back there. You're coming back with me, and you better behave. Your dad is furious with you. He wants to talk to you as soon as we are in Kirkcaldy. You can phone him!"

"What did I do? I don't know what I did wrong! I don't want to be in trouble!" I cried back at her. I do recall being on the phone to Dad who was still in Saudi Arabia. He was livid that I'd apparently 'screwed up'.

When we got to my sisters' house, I sat on the old brown couch in the living room. There were dirty dishes scattered about and the brown carpet needed a good hoover. Mum handed me the old cordless cream phone. It was tobacco from years of sitting in a smoker's house and the number keys were stiff to push. I dialled my Saudi telephone number and listened to the little clicks as the number processed. There wasn't a ringing sound, only two or three long dial tones before Dad picked up.

"Hello?" Dad answered.

"Dad? It's Mhairi." I started crying immediately.

"What did you do, you silly little girl? Do you realise the mess you've made? They don't want you back there because of your behaviour! You've ruined your education and now you'll have to come back here. Just you wait till you get here. You'll get a hot arse from me!" He was shouting so loudly down the phone he may as well have been standing in front of me.

It was all my fault: I hadn't behaved, I'd ruined a good opportunity. I just mumbled apologies for my bad behaviour through my sobs and sniffles and shut down there and then. I was eleven years old, but I was really nothing – nothing was left that had been there before, and what manifested itself over my silence was a completely different person. I was full of anger, and blamed myself for everything, especially for just lying there and taking it so weakly. I became the antithesis of who I had been before. There were times over the years when Mum and I would be reminiscing, and she'd ask me what had happened at school. It happened a few times.

"What happened, Mhairi? It was all so quick." She'd say.

"I don't know, Mum. You came for me, but I don't know why. You wantin' a cuppa?" I'd shut down the conversation, not yet ready to be open about what happened and not ready to ask why Mum suddenly appeared at the school to take me away. I had already chosen silence, and that was how it would stay until I was in my thirties.

CHAPTER 4

I finished the first year of high school in Saudi and stayed for all the second year. I'd been re-enrolled at my old school, Dhahran Academy. Mum and Dad never mentioned going back to the UK for school at first. Unsurprisingly, I didn't concentrate at school and my report cards often came back with 'satisfactory' or 'needs to try harder'.

I didn't care much for my peers either. I caught up with a few old friends who were still on the compound where we lived. I'd go out occasionally with my old rollerblading friends and some of us who were at swimming training together still met up at the pool and, though I still went to the usual birthday parties and outings, I never fully invested myself in friendships any more. I became protective of myself because I didn't want to get hurt and my trust in people was gone. If there was a hint of confrontation I either went into myself or lashed out. I remember there was a girl who I was friends with at school, Alice. We were good friends and had had sleepovers before I was sent to boarding school. One day at lunchtime at school, I wasn't feeling particularly chatty, and Alice was her usual happy, hair-flicking, bouncy self.

"Mhairi, there you are! Are you coming to the dome for lunch?" Alice asked in her Canadian twang.

"No, I'm just going to sit here and eat. It's nice and quiet here." I replied.

"Aw, come on! Don't be all moody and down. Come on!" She half bent down and held my arm to pull me up and I yanked my arm away and slapped her straight across the face.

"Leave me alone, Alice. I said no!" I picked up my lunchbox and stormed off. Our friendship ended after that and when my parents heard of it, I received the standard slapping across the bare bum that Dad so readily doled out.

I got back into swimming most days and, with some coaching from a lady on the compound, managed to gain multiple certificates and badges in different swimming strokes, water safety and lifesaving. The swimming gave me a focus and made me feel like I was achieving something. It was something I had to work hard for and only I could affect my results. When I wasn't swimming, I spent as much time as I could out on my bike or rollerblades, zooming around the roads for hours on end. I had flashbacks from the boarding school and would get anxious and fidgety just sitting in the house. Taking off on my rollerblades or my bike would give me a rush and would stop me overthinking things or going over things in my mind.

I also started my own little business looking after people's pets when they were away on holiday, so I always had something to look forward to. I would look after any pet from tiny little terrapins and quails to cats and dogs. These things kept me on a level of sorts and became a crutch that I relied upon because nothing ever got so bad that a furry or feathery hug and an hour or two in the sun wouldn't help ease. I spent less and less time with people around my own age. I didn't trust them at all and it was a far easier life having animal friends who couldn't hurt you.

We had a black and white cat of our own called Topsy. She was a big, cuddly girl who loved roaming about near our villa or cuddling up on my bed. If I saw her outside whilst I was cycling or rollerblading I'd shout to her, and she'd follow me back home. Gradually, it got to a point where I began to feel comfortable in myself. I went to school, spent as much time as I could with animals or outdoors and went on the odd outing with my parents. So long as I didn't waiver from my comfort zones, everything was settled.

Not long before my thirteenth birthday, I remember playing Scrabble with Mum and Dad one night. It was something we'd do once every couple of weeks when Dad's shifts meant he wasn't at work at night. The three of us would sit in the lounge around the oval rosewood coffee table with a glass of iced tea and some peanuts or cashews in a dish and play. We'd turn the television off and play some music. Dad liked Michael Jackson and Mum liked Eurythmics, so it was usually one of those that was put on. Dad always won, of course, coming up with some weird word like 'zaxes' or 'exequy' to use up the high-scoring letters. Still, I enjoyed the challenge, even if I did hate losing.

"We need to talk to you, Mhairi," Mum said one night after we'd finished. She looked serious. She got up and turned the volume down on the hi-fi. The buzz of the air conditioning seemed so loud now that the room was in silence. It was January, but it still hit the mid-twenties some nights.

"What's wrong?" I'd only had this sort of 'chat' once before, and it hadn't gone well. I started to worry at the serious look which had developed on Mum's face.

"It's about school. We need to think about where you'll finish high school. You know it can't be here," she said.

"Why not? Loads of people at school are staying on. Some are even going to the American school next door." I tried to brush it off, but I could feel the anxiety starting to bubble in my stomach.

"Yes, but we don't want you to go to the American school. You need to have a British education. It'll be better when you're trying to get into uni," Mum shot back.

"I might not go to uni though. I think I'll be fine staying here with you and going to school. I don't want to go back to Scotland."

I realised I wasn't going to get much more of a say when Dad pulled his reading glasses down his nose, sat forward, and peered over them at me sitting on the floor on the other side of the coffee table.

"Oh, we weren't thinking Scotland anyway," Dad piped up. "There's a good school we've heard about in Lancashire, near Blackpool. It looks and sounds lovely."

"I don't want to go back to boarding school. I'm not going back to boarding school. No way! You can't make me go. I don't know anyone there. I'll be all alone!"

"This isn't up for discussion, Mhairi," Dad said. "You need to go to school in the UK, and Mum and I are staying here. We've picked a good school that has good teachers and nice bedrooms for you. There's a caravan park just up the road which we're going to have a look at. It would be good to have a wee holiday place to stay and your Auntie Una has said she'll come up to see you at weekends and some holidays and stay in the caravan with you."

"Auntie Una? I hardly know her. I'm not going!" I started to raise my voice.

"You are going! That's an end to it. Next time we go back home we're going to visit the school and get the caravan so get used to the idea." Dad shouted back at me.

Dad's decision was final, and Mum's silence was confirmation. I was going and the chat was over.

***

In September 1997, from the front garden of my new boarding school in Lancashire, I watched tearfully as Mum and Dad drove out of the school grounds to their caravan less than a mile away. They had a couple of days left of their holiday before they went back to Saudi, but I wouldn't see them again until school broke up for Christmas. This school was bigger than my last boarding school and was mixed, rather than girls only. The girls' dorm block was a two-storey, purpose-built building, with green carpet and yellow walls in the halls. On the ground floor was the laundry, the matron's office, and her apartment. There were a couple of dorms for fourth years, but mainly single and double rooms for girls in the fifth and sixth years. On the first floor were four bedrooms which housed first to third-year girls. There were four of us to a bedroom, which had matching dark wood single wardrobes, bedside cabinets, and the familiar single metal-framed beds. The rooms were painted cream with dark blue, ridged carpets that were rough on your feet. There was a large white-tiled bathroom block at the end of the first-floor corridor which had four toilet cubicles, a bank of four sinks and four showers separated by shower curtains.

The girls in my dorm were nice enough and we got along okay. Annette's family were in Germany. She was a loud, brash girl who was about 5'9" and well-built with long brown hair. She looked much older than her fourteen years. Casey was as tall as Annette but was skinny and had a sleek dark brown bob. Her family were also in Germany. Beth was shorter at about 5'6" but was perfectly proportioned and her delicate face was framed with dyed blond hair that flowed down to the middle of her back. Her family had money and lived about an hour away from the school near Manchester. During the first year I was there, I did form some sort of relationship with them, albeit on a very basic level, but I never fully invested myself into becoming anybody's real friend. I always felt slightly on the outside, especially where material possessions were concerned.

"Look what I got from my mum for Christmas, girls!" Beth pulled out her sparkly light blue bottle of Angel by Thierry Mugler. "Obviously I got loads of other stuff too. We went shopping to Topshop. I'll show you my new jeans later."

"I got Cerruti perfume," Annette said. "A Kickers bag and I've got money back with me to go shopping for clothes."

"I got the Kickers I asked for and a new Kangol bag. Money obviously, and I went shopping to Topshop too. I bet we've got the same jeans, Beth!" Casey was rifling through her suitcase to pull her jeans out. "What about you, Mhairi?"

"I got a new rosewood jewellery box and some clothes for back in Saudi. I didn't really need anything for here. New stationery and some jewellery. I've left them at home though."

They compared their latest fashion statements, and I just went quietly about unpacking my stuff. I wasn't interested in having the best and most expensive things. A lot of the kids at the school were like that, but it just didn't interest me. I spoke to the other girls and boys as much as I needed to, to get by without being noticed too much. I largely kept myself to myself, which ultimately led to a reputation of me being unfriendly or anti-social.

"Are you coming to the woods?" Casey would ask. Out of the three of them, it would mostly be Casey that would still invite me to go places with her, Annette, and Beth.

"No, I think I'll just stay here and read," I'd reply.

"Suit yourself but if you change your mind, you know where we are. Beth's got a thing for Tom, so I think she's going to try and see if he'll go for a walk with her. See you later!"

Whilst little groups began to form, I'd often sit on my own in the common rooms watching the film that was on, or I'd be outside on the sports fields when the weather was nice, writing little poems or reading. Of course, there were times when I'd mingle with others, whether it was going into town on a Saturday or running about the school grounds in our free time, but by and large I was very much a loner. Sundays were the exception. We were made to go to church on a Sunday according to the school rules. You could only get out of it if you were too sick to walk, otherwise He would help you get over your ailments. Annette, Beth, Casey, and I hated going to church. We weren't the only ones either, but the four of us would stick together on the way down the hill to the town centre.

"Safeway, anyone?" Beth asked.

"Yes!" The other three of us would shout back.

"Right, quick, before we're seen," Beth said.

"Strawberry laces are mine!" That was Annette.

"Fizzy cola bottles for me today," Casey laughed.

"Dolly mixtures as per," I'd chime in.

We'd half walk, half run to Safeway and buy our sweets before hurrying back out and merging back in with the army of borders marching up the hill on the other side of town, towards the church. We weren't the only ones to do it, but it felt daring all the same. Then, we'd sit for two hours in church, daring each other to not make a noise without plastic packets of sweets, trying to stifle our giggles.

That was as social as I got. It allowed me to have a little bit of a feeling that I was included in a group of friends but being on my own was easier for me to cope with than getting too close to somebody like before. In my eyes, it was far better to be labelled as moody and a bit of an outcast than to put myself at any risk at all. I largely toed the line.

In June 1998, I was fourteen. I remember coming out of the dorm room late one Saturday or Sunday morning. Suddenly, a shooting pain like I had never felt before in my life ran through my pelvis. My toes started to tingle and then I began to feel nauseous. Within a couple of minutes, my whole body was shaking, and my eyesight fractured into coloured dots dancing all over the place. I couldn't stand up properly, and had to hold onto the wall for support as I edged my way along the corridor to the bathroom. I vomited, then span around to sit down for the deluge of diarrhoea that followed. I spent the next two days in bed with painkillers.

When I finally got up to go back to class, I was as weak as a kitten. The bleeding started not long after I had first vomited and was horrendously heavy from the start. I was worried about going back to class, which proved right because I leaked through my super tampon and my night-time sanitary towel to my school skirt on my first day back just before lunch. Nobody had explained to me about my periods starting. I didn't know how much blood I was going to lose. I had no idea how to use a tampon or a sanitary towel. I hadn't even spoken to the girls in the dorm about periods. The only reason I had towels and tampons at all was that I'd bought them at the shop on the caravan park one weekend because I thought they might come in handy. I'd read the instructions on the packets and done my best to fit everything where it was meant to go. This was my introduction to menstruation and the start of 'womanhood', a biological nightmare for me that would last almost two decades.

CHAPTER 5

My second year at the Lancashire boarding school was not unlike the first, only now I'd grown weary of being excluded and being the loner. My roommates were still friendly enough, but I was very much the odd one out. It started to eat away at me, and I became upset and angry again. All I wanted to do was go home. There was a makeshift phone box just outside the common room. It was basically a cupboard with a light and a payphone in it where I spent many evenings calling Mum and Dad, crying down the phone, begging them to take me home. I persisted, even though I knew that I would be staying exactly where I was.

When I went home for the Christmas holidays in 1998, I was nearing my fifteenth birthday. I wasn't looking forward to it because I knew the two weeks would fly by, and then I'd be packed off again. What was the point of even trying to broach the subject of not going back to school any more? To me, there wasn't one. That Christmas, I spent most of my time on my bike or in the pool, as was the case during all my holidays back home. One afternoon, I'd come back to the house, and for a reason I can't remember, an argument started between my parents and me. Mum raised her voice, then Dad started shouting, before I lost my temper and stomped upstairs to my room.

"And you can tell that standing beside you to fuck off!" I yelled at Mum, ignoring Dad next to her. I slammed the door, but he was coming right behind me. He came in, yanked my drawers down, bent me over his knee and smacked me. I wet myself all over his legs. I can't lie, it was a small victory having peed all down him.

"That is what that thinks of that," he said as he left the room. I composed myself and went out on my bike. I rode all around the compounds, went to the parks, and spent hours sitting in various quiet spots where I knew I wouldn't be found. By the time I returned home, it was well after sunset. Mum and Dad looked worried. I ignored Mum, walking straight past her. I walked right up to where Dad was sitting on the couch, looked down at him and for the first time in my life I stood up to him.

"You will never lay a hand on me again. If you do, I'll hit you back and then you'll never see me again." I was quiet and calm when I spoke. But every word was pronounced with a clarity that Dad could not ignore. I turned my back on him and walked away up the stairs towards my room before he got the chance to say anything, and he didn't follow me. The next night, we went out for dinner like nothing had ever happened. When the holidays were over, I went back to school with the realisation that I could only rely on myself from then on. I'd finally stood up to my dad and as scary as it had been it left me knowing that if I could stand up to him, I could stand up to anyone.

***

The next holidays were Easter 1999. I didn't go back to Saudi; instead, Mum and Dad came to their caravan near to my school. One day we went for a drive to a little village called Elswick, about twenty minutes away. We parked in the village hall car park, and when we all got out of the car, Dad pointed over the road to some brand-new red-brick houses that were being built.

"What do you think?" he asked.

"They're nice. Why are we here?" I answered.

"We're going to have a look at one, and if we like it, we might just get one, eh Joyce?" He glanced over at Mum, who beamed approvingly.

"Yes! You're coming home? Can I come here too?" I asked.

"Yep. Well, Mum will come back from Saudi first and then I'll come back not long after but, yes, you can go to school every day from home."

I was so happy I started to cry. I couldn't believe this was happening. Dad hugged me first and I squeezed him tightly. "Thank you," I said, before pulling Mum into the hug. "Thank you both so much. This is amazing."

The house we viewed was the first of eight houses on the road. I stood beside Mum and Dad, looking up at the red brick house with white window frames. It had white scalloped roof edging and a lovely big bay window like the one we had in our old house in Kirkcaldy. There was a drive to the left of the house that had a double gate leading up the side of the house, and there was a small square of grass in front of the window.

"This is the show house," Dad said. "It's number one. The one that we might get is number three, down there." He pointed to the third house down that had scaffolding built up all round it and was just all dirt and stones surrounding it. "It's exactly the same as that one will be, but we will buy all our own furniture and choose nice carpets and curtains."

We went in the front door and through a little square porch to a glass-panelled door that led to the main house. There was a study to the left.

"Aw Mum, you'll be able to have your own office space. You can get nice bookshelves for all your books and ornaments," I said.

"That would be lovely. I could just imagine the computer sat in there whilst I look over the fields with a cuppa. Might need to get an updated computer, though." She glanced at Dad, who gave her a little wink.

The stairs were next to the study, so we ventured up to see the four bedrooms. At the top of the stairs was a double linen cupboard. To the right was the master bedroom with ensuite shower room and another single bedroom. To the left was a double bedroom, a single bedroom, and a bathroom with its own bath. I headed left to the double bedroom. The window looked out over the back garden and onto the garage. Directly opposite the bedroom was the bathroom.

"Hey. Mum? Dad? Can I have this bedroom? I love it." They both came into the room beside me. "Would that be okay?" I asked.

"I think that would be okay with us." Dad said, smiling. "It seems like you have your own bathroom, too."

"My own bathroom? Is that really my own bathroom?" I asked.

"Unless I'm in the bath," Mum said. "I like my baths but when I'm not, it's all yours."

"This is amazing. I can just see my bed in here with a nice matching wardrobe and chest of drawers. Not having to share it with three other people. And to be able to go to the bathroom whenever I want and not have to queue for a shower. This is the best," I said.

We went back downstairs where there was a little toilet room on the other side of the staircase. Opposite that door was the door to the living room. We went into the room and stood for a few seconds, taking in the space.

"It's amazing, Allan," Mum said. "Look at that fireplace. All dark wood surround that will match our coffee tables perfectly. I like the floral tiles too. But we'll have a look and see what they've got in the catalogue if we like it."

"Look at you, picking décor already," Dad laughed. "It's pretty special, though. Look at the view from here. Just open fields and greenbelt apparently, so there can't be any houses built there for a good few years anyway."

"I think Topsy will love the fields. You are bringing her home with you, aren't you?" I asked. I couldn't imagine not having our little Saudi cat enjoy all the lush green fields to run about in.

"Of course, she's coming back with us. She'll need to go into quarantine for six months but we're not leaving her in Saudi." Mum said.

"Just think of her all curled up in the winter in front of the fire." I said. I turned to the left and through an archway that split the room in two. The front half was the living room, and the back half was the dining room with double sliding doors that led out to the back garden. "Aw, just think of this in the summer. We could have a few barbecues and sit out on the patio."

"You going to cook it?" Dad asked.

"Pretty sure I could give it a go if you don't mind taking a risk with sausages. What's through here?"

I turned left again and went through a door which led us into a large kitchen with room for a table and chairs, and there was a separate utility room with a washing machine and a tumble drier fitted in.

"Well, this is rather nice," Mum said. What a decent size."

"I do like it," Dad said. "There's a fridge/freezer built in here too, and a dishwasher."

"A dishwasher?" I asked. "You have no idea how happy that makes me. No hassle to clean up after dinner. That garage out there is massive, by the way. You'd get two cars in there."

"Good," Dad said. "We'll probably need two eventually. There looks like there's room for a chest freezer, too. For extra bits and bobs if we have a house full."

"The whole place is amazing. I love it. Can we move here?" I asked.

"Oh, your dad and I will need to talk about it," Mum said. "But I do love it. It's got everything we could ever want."

We all loved it and when we left and got back in the car, Dad drove for about twenty minutes through little country lanes, admiring all the little villages that we went through. He turned back towards Elswick and then stopped in a layby that was far enough away from the house we had just viewed to be out of sight, but close enough that we could look at the eight proud buildings from afar.

"Should we buy it?" Dad asked Mum.

"Can we afford it?" she said.

"Yes. If Mhairi's not boarding, and we both have jobs, we'll be fine." Dad replied.

"Then let's do it. Let's buy it!" Mum said.

"That okay with you?" Dad said as he turned to me.

"That's fine with me. Yes please!" I replied.

"Okay then," he said.

We drove back to the show home, and Dad signed the papers there and then. I went back to school to see the end of year out. At the end of term, I packed up all my things, knowing it was the last time I'd ever set foot in a boarding school dorm. I couldn't get out of the place quick enough.

***

We spent the summer unpacking and making our new house a home. Mum and Dad had already chosen the cream carpets to be laid throughout the house as they had been back in England for a couple of weeks before I had finished school. The custom-made green floral curtains were on order, as was the green floral three-piece-suite to match the curtains.

"Can I pick my furniture and curtains for my bedroom please?" I asked them both when I got back from school. They'd bought me a single bed that had another bed underneath for if I ever had friends around. I just liked the idea that I could make up a double bed when I felt like it in my spacious bedroom.

"Yes, you can," Mum said. "You want to have a look through the catalogue?" She handed me the thick, heavy booklet and I thumbed through it until I reached the bedroom furniture section. I looked through the pages.

"I like this set here. But in the blue, not the pink." I said. I'd chosen a wardrobe, bedside cabinet and large chest of drawers that had a light pine frame and cornflower blue drawer and door fronts. "Do you think I could get the blue bookshelf to match? All my books are here from Saudi, and I'd like them in my room."

"I don't think that would be a problem," Mum said. "What about curtains?"

"I like these blue and yellow ones here." I pointed out the curtains which had alternating blue and yellow vertical stripes on them.

"They're absolutely fine," Mum said. "I'll get them ordered for you."

By the end of the summer, we had looked through countless catalogues, choosing furniture and soft furnishings for each room. Time flew by but I wasn't dreading going back to school because all I had to do was get on the bus in the morning and come back in the afternoon. I had a big year ahead with my GCSEs due in May 2000. The first term, from September to December 1999, was spent studying for our mock exams in the following January. It was a busy term so there wasn't much time for socialising or hanging about aimlessly with each other that had been the normal in previous years.

Once the mock exams were over in February 2000 it was a little different. There was more spare time or, as teachers liked to call it, study periods. My previous two years as a boarder, staying at arm's length from everybody, had done me no favours at all, because now I was nobody's friend. Cliques had been formed, bonds made, and outsiders were not only unwelcome but targets, and I was one of those targets. I didn't have the 'safety' of being a boarder either. Being a boarder seemed to give you a little immunity as it was recognised that your family, and therefore your access to money, was limited. Now, as a day pupil, I had that so-called access to money and therefore had the expectation from other kids that I would have the big-named clothes, the latest accessories and a certain amount of cash floating about in my schoolbag. Everything I wore, down to my underwear, was scrutinised by the rich kids.

I was an easy target for name-calling because I was Scottish, didn't wear labels, and I was a chubby size twelve in a changing room full of toned, tanned eights and tens. It didn't help that my second name was Hutt, so the 'Jabba the Hutt' jokes were inevitable. I'd occasionally snap back with a loud tirade of abuse which was greeted by laughter, or a parody of my accent, followed by a telling-off from a teacher who'd heard me shouting. It was hell, and I hated every minute of it. It didn't help that one of the girls who joined in with these jibes was the deputy head's daughter. She'd stand there with the other girls who would quietly mock me.

"Oh, look there's Jabba with her CKs." Rachel whispered to her posse just loud enough for me to hear. "Where's your haggis, Jabba?" She jibed in a fake Scottish twang.

"Her Calvin Klein pants?" Jess giggled.

"No!" Laughed Rachel. "Her chubby knickers." There was a chorus of sniggers around the changing room.

"Leave me the fuck alone. Shut up!" I yelled back. Then an ominous figure appeared in the doorway.

"Mhairi? Why are you shouting. My office now! Your temper needs to be kept in check." Miss Atkinson said. I dutifully followed her to her office and explained the situation.

"I'm sorry I shouted but they won't leave me alone," I said.

"Look I'll have to talk to the other teachers about this and see what we can do. That means talking to Fiona's mum, Mrs Bartlet, seeing as she's deputy head. Leave it with me."

A few days went by, and I was called in to Mrs Bartlet's office.

"Mhairi," she said, "Miss Atkinson spoke to me about the incident in the changing rooms the other day. I've spoken to Fiona, and she paints a very different picture from you. Apparently, you were the antagonist. She said you were quite rude to Rachel and Jess and then began shouting, which is when Miss Atkinson came in because she heard you."

"That's not true," I replied. "They were making fun of my weight and my underwear because it wasn't designer."

"Look, just keep a low profile, okay. Fiona is my daughter, and she won't get in trouble. Given you were the one shouting, I'm inclined to believe her version of events. Don't let me hear any more of this or it will go on your record formally, okay?" Mrs Bartlet got up and opened the door. "Off you go. Don't let me see you again."

I left the room with a silent 'fuck you'. I stopped going to school after that.

***

I pretended everything was normal to Mum and Dad. I'd say bye and pretend to go to get the school bus in the morning but instead of doing that I'd nip across the road and wait behind the village hall from where I could see the house, until they left and then I'd let myself back into the house. I would occasionally go into school but when I did go in, I was so far behind with my schoolwork that I didn't know half the stuff they were teaching. I nearly got caught a couple of times when Mum or Dad came home, but I hid in the garage until they left again. Teachers would leave messages on the house phone, but I'd delete them before either Mum or Dad could play them back. The school sent letters to the house that I ripped up before Mum or Dad saw them. Inevitably, I did get caught eventually. One of the teachers had managed to find out where Mum worked and telephoned her. That night, when Mum and Dad came home, we had a massive argument.

"You stupid little girl," Dad roared at me. "Do you know what your Mum and I gave up to come back to the UK? You, stupid, ungrateful little bitch." He was physically shaking with anger; so much so that his glasses wouldn't stay on the end of his nose where he usually placed them to peer over them whilst dishing out lectures. He had to remove them completely. I found that a little humorous.

"Mhairi, this isn't funny," Mum said. She was going red and, far from shouting, she was calm, clear, and quiet. "We've sacrificed a lot to come back home so you could come out of boarding school. You need to go to school and get your exams done."

"Oh, I'm so sorry for the sacrifices the two of you had to make! God forbid I've mucked your lives up." I said.

"You are not going to throw your life away like this. You'll get back to school even if I have to drive you there myself every day," Dad said.

"I'm not going back. I'm done." I said.

"You'll get back and get your exams done while you're under my roof, young lady, or …"

"Or what, Dad?" I yelled. "Or you'll smack me? You'll kick me out? I'll tell you what your problem is. You've spent years not having Lesley, Sharon or me around. You shipped me off to boarding school at ten years old and left your other two teenage daughters with two pensioners. You wouldn't know how to deal with any of us anyway. All you did was suit yourself. You wanted to be in Saudi and fuck what your children needed or wanted. You're just a selfish arsehole. You don't know how to be a dad!"

"Get out! Get out of my house now!" he roared.

"With pleasure," I said. I ran upstairs and phoned Laura, a girl I'd become friends with, in the village.

"Laura, my parents have kicked me out. Do you think I could stay at yours for a few nights until I sort something out?" I asked.

"Oh my god, are you okay? I'll ask my parents. They should be fine with it. Hang on a minute. I held the phone to my ear with my shoulder whilst I hastily shoved some clothes and toiletries into a holdall. "Mhairi? That's fine. Just for a few nights though, okay?"

"Thank you so much. I'll be over in about half an hour." I replied. I finished packing my holdall and walked down the stairs, into the kitchen where Mum and Dad were standing talking to each other. I walked straight past them without a word and walked out the back door, slamming it shut on my way out.

The next morning, I phoned my sister, Lesley. Lesley was now twenty-two, and she had just qualified as a nurse. She'd moved to Blackpool from Kirkcaldy the year before and had a baby, my little niece, Cerys, who was a little over four months old.

"Lesley, it's Mhairi. Please can I come and live with you?" I pleaded.

"What's wrong?" She replied.

"Fucking Mum and Dad, that's what's wrong. Dad kicked me out. We had a massive row because they found out I was skipping school. I was getting a hard time from a group of girls and couldn't hack it any more. Dad went mental so I told him a few home truths, mainly that he abandoned us all and was a shit dad. He didn't like that very much and kicked me out," I said. I could her a little giggle down the phone.

"Oh well, you didn't lie to him. Truth hurts, I suppose. Yes, you can come and stay but, Mhairi, I work full time and I have Cerys, remember? You'll need to get a job and help me in the house and help look after Cerys. Okay?" She spoke.

"Perfect," I replied. I was grateful she had a spare room and was going to take me in, and I promised to help her with Cerys.

CHAPTER 6

When I moved into Lesley's, I wrote to my headmaster at school and explained my home situation to him. I told him how I was now living with my sister and young baby and that it would be difficult for me to go back to school. I also explained to him about the bullying that had been going on and that that was the reason I had stopped going to school in the first place. All I could do after that was wait, but for what I didn't know.

In the meantime, I absolutely doted on Cerys. She was such a calm baby and I loved how she used to snuggle into my neck and fall asleep so easily. I'd sing to her or read to her when she was awake and when I wasn't doing that, I was giving her a running commentary on whatever I was doing. I'm sure I bored her rotten at times.

Whilst staying with Lesley I got a job at a fast-food place at nights and, while Lesley was working at the hospital during the day, I'd look after Cerys, dressing her up in cute wee outfits and taking her for days out down to Blackpool beach or trips to the shops. I used to love it when people would come up and admire her, and I never used to correct people when they asked how old 'my baby' was. The bond we had was loving and trusting, certainly for me, given that Cerys wasn't even a year old yet. It was during this time I decided how much I wanted a baby at some point. That feeling of complete love for someone so tiny, and knowing it was my job to care and nurture her, was something I felt I could so easily take to, despite feeling I hadn't been given that same chance with my parents. It was the first time in my life that I'd thought of becoming a parent, but I knew it was something I wanted to do. Cerys was the beginning of that, and at this point in my life she became my main focus. My only focus, perhaps. I'd finished with school, and I'd had enough of my parents. For once, I was doing my own thing, and holding tight to that little bit of happiness that was my baby niece.

One day, when I'd only been in Blackpool for a month or so, I was out in the shopping centre with Cerys. I saw a girl I recognised from school, Felicity. She hadn't been one of the bullies, so I felt confident enough to call over to her. She turned round at hearing her name and I waved. She looked over for a moment and I called again and waved, walking over to her. She looked at Cerys then up at me.

"What have you been up to?" I noted a little smirk on her face.

"Oh! Ha ha! This is my niece, Cerys. I'm staying with my sister just now. Moved out …"

"Mhairi look, my mum said I really shouldn't hang around people like you. Nothing personal, you understand. I need to go." And she turned and walked quickly away. To this day I have no idea why she said that nor what 'people like me' was supposed to mean. Whether she believed Cerys was mine or not I don't know, but it was the one and only time I'd told anybody that didn't know who we were, who Cerys was. Normally I liked to play along if Cerys got attention. She was a cute baby so if people thought she was mine, I didn't feel the need to correct them. I felt so small in that instant, as Felicity turned and walked away. All I could do was hurry home, with tears running down my face. What had she told her mum about me that would lead her to that conclusion? Clearly something had been gossip-worthy. Even though I was still only sixteen, I realised just how much I hated gossips and liars.

There were times I'd look after Cerys not out of necessity whilst Lesley was at work, but to let Lesley away for a break for a few days. One of the times I looked after Cerys, Lesley was in Newcastle with friends. I booked some time off work, and it was like a little holiday for me and Cerys to spend some time together. By this time, she was crawling all over the place, so I had to have eyes on her all the time. She never went very far though.

One afternoon, I took my eye off the ball. Cerys was crawling around the living room, and I was in the kitchen getting her bottles in the steriliser and tidying up. I made myself a cup of tea and took it through to the living room. Without thinking, I put it down on a ledge on the fireplace that was barely a foot off the ground. I walked back through to the kitchen and went to grab a tea towel from the worktop when I heard the most awful blood-curdling scream I ever heard in my life. Cerys! I ran through to the living room and saw the teacup on the floor, and Cerys writhing around beside it. I scooped her up in one arm, somehow managed to grab my phone and ran up the stairs to the bathroom. I had a long, white linen skirt on, perfect to soak with cold water and try to stem the burning that Cerys was feeling; I stepped straight into the bath and turned on the cold tap on, yanked my skirt off and shoved it under the tap. Then I wrapped Cerys in it and phoned an ambulance. I was bawling my eyes out when they arrived just a few minutes later. I couldn't believe I'd been so stupid and hurt Cerys. I managed to phone Lesley while I was in the ambulance,

"Lesley! I'm so sorry. I'm in an ambulance with Cerys. I left my fresh cup of tea on the fireplace ledge, and she pulled it over herself." I cried down the phone to her.

"Oh shit! "Is she okay? How bad is it?" she asked.

"It's not bad. The paramedics said she'll be okay. Just precautionary to go to the hospital. We should be home in a couple of hours. I am so sorry." I said.

"Mars, it's okay." She'd called me Mars. That was Lesley's pet name for me. It meant that things really were okay.

"These things happen. Please don't worry. The main thing is that Cerys is okay. Just phone me and let me know when you are home all right?" She was so nice about it. When I got off the phone, one of the paramedics spoke to me.

"You really did good, you know. That was a scary situation, and most people would panic. The fact you acted so quick with your skirt in the bathtub had probably saved Cerys from having serious burn damage. Accidents happen, love. She'll be fine," he said. After spending hours at the hospital, I eventually got Cerys back home. I cradled her and apologised over and over. I still feel guilty about it now. For all my good intentions, I was still young.

When Lesley returned, she told me she was pregnant again, and the new baby was due at the end of January. It was September by then, so she only had four months to go before there were two babies around. I still felt guilty about the tea incident with Cerys. I felt that I hadn't been careful enough. In my mind I knew that looking after two babies would be far too difficult for me to cope with so, I decided the time had come for me to move out of Lesley's flat. It broke my heart to leave Cerys, but I knew I couldn't stay.

***

I ended up back in Kirkcaldy, staying with a cousin who was good enough to take me in. I only stayed a few months. I started to work at the local bingo hall and made a few girlfriends. One of them, Sarah, was looking to move into a flat, so we decided to move in together. We managed to get a place down near the seafront. At that time, The Links in Kirkcaldy was well known for drug users and discarded paraphernalia. Still, if you kept yourself to yourself, you usually weren't bothered by anybody. The flat was in a block of six three-bedroomed maisonettes, with each flat costing a grand total of £350 per month to rent in 2001. It was affordable on our basic bingo wages and suited Sarah and I for our bus journey to work, and it was only a couple of minutes' walk into the town centre. Things were okay for a couple of months. We managed to pay the bills and have food in the house, and always made sure we had money for our three-litre bottle of cider, quarter bottle of Grouse, and cigarettes for the weekend.

One night in February, after work, Sarah introduced me to her friend Michael. She organised a lift back to the flat from him as it was bad snow and the buses had stopped running. He was an unassuming, skinny guy that was about 5'9". He had a skinhead, and a long, oblong face – the type that always looks like a sad puppy. He wore straight-cut jeans, white trainers, and a white polo T-shirt. He was only a year or so older than me and not my usual type, but we hit it off anyway. He had his own car, liked a laugh, and didn't put pressure on me for anything beyond the friendship that we struck up. Even so, he soon became a permanent fixture in the flat, although we never made our relationship a formal one of being a couple and it never went past the casual sex stage. The weekends were a blur of alcohol. We had parties every weekend where we got drunk and stoned with the neighbours from the surrounding flats. But, once cocaine started appearing in the house, I knew I had to think about getting out of the flat. I was fine with casual cannabis use but I didn't want to move on to anything harder. Sarah and I had no savings so we couldn't afford to get another flat.

"Why don't we go and stay with my mum and stepdad?" Sarah said. "My old room is plenty big, and it's a double bed so we could both sleep in there."

"Are you sure they'd be okay with it? I don't really know them. Would be handy till we saved up some cash to get another flat, though," I replied.

"Aye, they'll be fine."

And that was that. One phone call later, Sarah's stepdad agreed to come with a van the next day to take us back to his house to stay. We didn't even warn the landlord. We just upped and left, posting the keys through the letterbox.

For the first month, it was fun living at Sarah's house. Her mum, stepdad, sister and two brothers were all living in the house, which made for a busy, fun atmosphere. The boys would help Sarah's stepdad outside with DIY, while the girls helped her mum with laundry, cooking and cleaning. I didn't mind, even if it was a bit regimented. There were set mealtimes, set shared bath times, allocated family time and rules were made to be followed. It wasn't unusual to hear one of the girls or boys in tears, having been smacked by their stepdad for disobeying an order or missing a timeslot. I made sure I kept to the rules to avoid the worst.

One evening I was walking up the stairs at about 7pm with my towel, ready to jump into Sarah's used bathwater. She hadn't shouted me up like she usually did, so I thought she'd just forgotten. Halfway up the stairs, I saw her come out of her mum and stepdad's bedroom, looking flustered. She turned her head away, and ran down the stairs into our room. The bedroom door was left open a crack; I saw Sarah's stepdad sitting on the edge of the bed, putting his trainers on. I felt a bit strange. I walked into the bathroom, shutting the door behind me, wedging the hand towel under the door, which had no lock. It was the quickest wash I think I ever had. I practically ran back down the stairs and into my room. Sarah looked no better than when I'd last seen her. Her eyes were red from crying.

"What happened, hun?" I asked. "Are you okay?"

"It doesn't matter," she sniffed.

"Please, Sarah. What's wrong? You can tell me anything, you know."

"Please don't say anything. It's John. I thought when I moved out, it wouldn't ever start again, but it has."

"What has?"

"The dry humping."

"The what?"

"The dry humping!"

I had no idea what dry humping was, but it was obvious that Sarah was talking about something awful. She had never opened up to me about anything like this before. It turned out that before we moved into the flat, John had been making Sarah sit on top of him, or vice versa, and pretend to have sex with him. They were both fully clothed, but all the actions were carried out and the result for him was the same. It stopped when she moved out and hadn't happened again until that night. I hugged her until she fell asleep through her tears and sniffles. In the morning, it was still playing on her mind.

"Don't tell anyone, please. I couldn't stand what he'd do if he found out."

"I won't, Sarah, but we need to get a flat as quickly as possible and get out of here, okay?"

"Okay."

A week later, on one of my days off work, John asked me to go with him to his brother's house near Dunfermline, about twenty minutes away. I reluctantly agreed and got in the van with him, sitting as close to the passenger door as I possibly could. There was a strange silence, as if he knew I knew what had been going on with him and Sarah, but he said nothing. I said nothing. We arrived at his brother's house, and I silently followed him in. His brother was there alone.

"Hi Nigel,. just poppin' in to introduce you to Mhairi. She's Sarah's workmate, and they're back staying with us for a while." John grinned at his brother, and I suddenly felt uneasy. I could feel Nigel's eyes fumbling all over me, with John's eyes not far behind. I was wearing beige cargo pants that were tight on my bum, and a cropped cream vest, but I never felt more naked and on display. Neither of them spoke to me.

"Oh, this is Mhairi. I see what you mean." He followed this with a disturbing chuckle. "I was wondering when I'd meet her. Fits in nicely, does she?"

Where do I fit in, Nigel? I don't like this at all.

"Oh aye. Very nicely. I think we're nearly there anyway, ha ha."

Nearly where, John? What are you talking about? Don't even think about making me like Sarah!

I started to feel really uncomfortable and couldn't wait to get out of there. Luckily, it was just an introductory visit, so we were only there about fifteen minutes. I silently followed John back to the van and sidled up to the passenger door for the journey home.

"You can come closer to me, you know? I won't bite unless you tell me to."

I nearly screamed. He was going to make me like Sarah, forcing me to satisfy his lewd fantasies. I didn't get a chance to reply.

"When we're in the house, Mhairi, I'd like it if you keep dressing like you are just now. Wear things that cling to your arse and show off your figure. It suits you and I like it."

He put his hand on my right thigh and smiled. I didn't reply. I looked at him, hoping he wouldn't see how close I was to tears. We got home, and I got out the van as quickly as I dared. In the three days that followed, I wore the baggiest clothes I could find and stayed mostly in the bedroom. He would always be hanging about outside the bathroom when I was washing or coming into the bedroom unannounced. I couldn't stand it. I told Sarah what happened, and she seemed nonchalant.

"I was wondering when he'd start on you," Sarah said to me.

"Could you not have warned me about this, Sarah? A heads up might have been nice. I never would have stayed here if I knew this was happening. For your sake as well as mine."

"I'm used to it. I hate it but what can I do?"

"Report him?"

"What would that do? My mum would hate me …"

"She knows?"

"Yeah, she knows. Everyone does."

"You bitch! You brought me here knowing this would happen. I'm done. You can all go to hell. I'm off!"

I stormed through to the kitchen and got a roll of black bags. I flung everything I could find of mine into the bags, not caring what was clean or dirty, or doing my usual careful checking that I wasn't breaking anything. It didn't take long. Three black bags later, I was outside the house, getting in a taxi to Nana and Papa's house just on the other side of Kirkcaldy. I didn't know what I was going to say, or how I would explain my sudden appearance, but I knew I just needed familiarity and comfort.

I knocked on Nana and Papa's door and waited patiently for one of them to toddle through from the kitchen, along the hall and to the front door. Nana answered the door, neat as she always was in her navy calf-length skirt, nude tights, navy court shoes with an inch block heel, a fine knit jumper, and her pinnie, tied neatly at the waist.

"Hello, Mhairi. It's been a while. Come in and I'll put the kettle on," Nana said. That was always her first port of call, the kettle. Over the next couple of hours, I tried to explain to Nana and Papa what had happened, but in truth I wanted to spare them the details. They were in their eighties and didn't need the stress of trying to navigate my latest woes.

"Just call your mum and dad, Mhairi. I think it's maybe time you go home. They do worry about you, you know," Nana said. So, I did. I rang home and spoke to Dad.

"Dad, I want to come home. Please can you come and get me at Nana's?"

I was crying before I could stop myself. I felt like I was back in boarding school, pleading with him to let me come home and just waiting for his refusal. I was petrified but I had made the dreaded 'something bad has happened, please can I come home' phone call, and to my relief Dad said he would be up to get me and take me home. I waited a long two days before Dad arrived to stay overnight then take me back home. When I saw him, I rushed over and gave him a tearful hug. Relief washed over me because for the first time in my life, I had begged my parents to help me and finally, they had come and rescued me. I didn't feel alone any more.

About an hour after he arrived, Dad took his packet of menthol cigarettes out of his pocket, took one out and went out to the garden to sit on the little walled-in flowerbed. I waited a few seconds, took one of my own menthol cigarettes out of my packet which was in my jacket in the hall and went and sat beside him on the wall. He looked at me, surprised, as I lit my cigarette. I laughed at him and gave him a nudge.

"Like father, like daughter I'm afraid. I much preferred your Yves-Saint-Laurent ones in Saudi though," I teased him.

"You little bugger! You must have been fourteen or so when you started then?" he replied.

"I started pinching them off you when I was twelve. Naughty me. No lectures though, eh?" I said.

"I think we're past that point, don't you?" He smiled warmly at me. "Anything else to get off your chest?"

"Yes, actually. I've got tattoos, and I'll probably get more. While I've been away from home, I've been through a lot, and I've had to deal with it alone. I managed fine up until now. I've worked hard and looked after myself, paid my own way and I haven't asked anyone for anything. So, I'll do the same when I'm home with you and Mum. I'll get a job, pay my way, and help around the house but I am my own person and I'll ultimately make my own decisions. I'll respect your rules if they're reasonable, but you need to respect me too. Okay?" I spoke calmly to Dad, and he listened.

"That's fair enough," he replied. "I'm senior nurse at a nursing home close to the house. We need staff so if you don't mind having me as your boss then there's a job there if you want it and can do it. I'll just need to speak to the manager of the home first."

"Working with you? That should be interesting but, okay, deal." I said.

Our massive argument the previous year wasn't even mentioned, as if it hadn't even happened. Instead, there was mutual respect and honesty. We now knew exactly where we stood with each other, and for the first time in my life I felt as though I had parents I could rely on.

CHAPTER 7

True to his word, Dad spoke to the manager of the care home where he worked, and I was asked to go in for an informal chat. A few days later, early in September 2001, I started work as a care assistant with my dad as my boss. I worked with my dad a lot, and he taught me how to care for the residents like only he could. He had such a lovely manner with everybody, a unique sense of humour, and a wicked grin that nobody could resist. But more than that, he taught me how to properly care for somebody, to make sure that their every need was met. From helping to get the residents out of bed in the morning to get washed and dressed, helping to feed them, having a sing song, and reminiscing to making them comfortable in their dying minutes and hours – he taught me everything, and, like father, like daughter, I took to it with natural flair, and I loved going into work.

When we both worked together on the same sections, we had a laugh with the residents who were up to it, and shared more tender moments with those who were gravely ill. It was only two months into my time at the care home that I started working towards NVQ certificates in care with my workmate Natasha. Natasha was broad Glaswegian but had moved to Blackpool a few years earlier. I think we found common ground in that we were two of three Scottish people in the home. Dad suggested we apply to go to university to pursue a nursing diploma, which we both did. I filled in the forms with Dad by my side, and sent them off, wondering when I'd hear back. When I wasn't at work, I was at home helping Mum and Dad with mundane chores: keeping the house clean or taking my beautiful yellow Labrador, Glen, for long walks and playing with him in the garden. I was settled, for the first time in a long time.

In January 2002 I received the long-awaited university letter telling me I'd been accepted for an interview for my nursing diploma course. I was delighted with myself. It was the first time I'd achieved something this big, and Mum and Dad were proud of me too. It was all I could think about, and I told the residents at the nursing home, who all congratulated me and told me I'd do great.

On March 19, 2002, I put on a brand-new navy-blue suit, which had flared trousers and a subtle sparkle. I ironed a new cream blouse – picking up an iron was a miracle for me. I met Natasha at the university, and we nervously held each other's hands going into the large hall which had a waiting area with a table and a young woman sitting behind it, checking the interviewees in. There were twenty chairs set in four rows of five where we were sent to sit and wait for our names to be called. The rest of the hall was sectioned off into cubicles by blue curtains akin to those you would find on a hospital ward. Natasha and I both got called to our interviewers at the same time. I followed my interviewer, a stout, serious looking woman with dark brown hair pulled up into a tight ponytail which swished back and forth against the collar of her black blouse.

"Why do you want to be a nurse?" She asked first.

"My dad's been a nurse for well over twenty years and I work with him. He taught me how to look after people. If I could be half the nurse that he is then I'd be doing well. I just want to look after people and make sure they get the care they need," I replied.

"Okay, and what do you think you could bring to the role?" she continued.

"I'm caring and respectful. I'm a good listener, too. Mostly, though, I spent a lot of my younger years feeling like I wasn't cared about, and I wouldn't want anybody to feel like that if they were under my care." I answered confidently, but I was so frightened I was coming out with rubbish answers. There were so many questions, and my answers became a blur of words but, somehow, I got to the end of the interview unscathed. The interviewer smiled at me, and I relaxed a little.

"Well done. I know it can seem a bit daunting getting asked so many questions. I'm pleased to tell you that I'd like to offer you a place on the course!" She said.

"What? I'm in? Oh my god! Thank you. Thank you so much!"

I got up out of my seat and went and shook her hand, then went to the waiting room to wait for Natasha. I'd only gone and done it. My hard work had paid off, and what made it even better was Natasha got accepted on the spot too. We were like giddy schoolgirls that day. All the way back to the home, we were laughing and screaming, not quite believing that we'd managed to get into university. Everyone was so pleased for us, nobody more so than my dad and mum. Natasha and I promised each other we'd go out on the Saturday coming to celebrate, wearing our interview outfits. The day before I went out with Natasha, Dad handed me a present.

"Just a wee thing to say congratulations. I'm so proud of you," he said.

I gave him a massive hug and started crying. It was all I'd ever wanted to hear from my dad, and I'd finally heard it. I opened the gift.

"I know they're your favourite just now," he smiled.

He'd bought me a Westlife CD. What a great dad. He was right, they were my favourite but, in a move only a father could make, he'd bought me a Westlife tribute act CD. I didn't have the heart to tell him. I still have it, and I smile every time I see it.

Dad dropped me off at Natasha's flat on the Saturday afternoon. We spent hours getting ready to go out, taking our time putting our make-up on, having drinks between foundation and bronzer, eyeshadow, and mascara and, because neither of us owned a pair of straighteners, we ironed our hair under a towel on the ironing board. It worked well enough at the time. Before we knew it, we were half-cut and out in the centre of Blackpool. We had a couple of drinks in one pub before moving on to Brannigans, our favourite haunt, which always had a decent tribute act on. That night, it was a tribute act to Jake and Elwood themselves: The Blues Brothers. Our tipple was Smirnoff Ice, which we drank like juice, suffering the consequences later. One of our other mates drank pints, and Natasha and I usually managed to sink three Smirnoff Ices to their one pint. The good old days of not knowing what you were ingesting.

Natasha and I took it in turns going to the bar, and it must have been three or four rounds in when it was my turn to go up. I left the dancefloor and walked up to the bar to wait to be served. It was busy enough that I couldn't physically touch the bar yet, there were two rows of people in front of me, so I had about a five-minute wait before being served. Once I had our drinks in my hands, I turned to walk back to where Natasha was dancing on her own. I looked to my left, only to do a double-take and meet a pair of beautiful hazel eyes. They were piercing right through me. He was with two other men, but he was the one who stood out. He had jet-black hair, a short, back and sides, with subtle spikes on top, not quite hiding the slightly receding sides of his widow's peak. He had a chiselled jawline, which was covered with a dark five o'clock shadow. He was wearing dark trousers, and a blue-and-white striped shirt, with white collar and cuffs, his clothes just fitting enough to hint at a well-looked-after body, but loose enough to keep you guessing. He smiled at me, showing off his perfectly straight, white teeth. I attempted to smile back, instead getting a nervous jolt right through me. I put my head down and hurried back to Natasha.

My heart was racing by the time I got to her, but she was too busy dancing to notice. I handed her a bottle and joined her. For I few minutes, I looked around, trying not to be too obvious, but I'd lost sight of the man. I felt a tap on my shoulder. I turned round, and there he was. My heart started to pound. He was even more beautiful up close. Perfect skin, a gleaming smile, and those eyes up close, just inviting me to get lost in them. He smelled delicious – woody and spicy, but in a soft way.

"Hi, I'm Nick," he said, leaning into my ear. I felt his warm breath against my neck.

"Mhairi. Nice to meet you." His mates had turned their backs and were talking to each other, while Natasha was dancing with some randoms in the middle of the floor.

"Fancy a dance?" he asked.

"Yeah, that would be good."

We danced together while the band finished their set. He was twirling me round, pulling me close, and looking right into my eyes then pushing me back out again and we were both laughing and mouthing along to the words. When the band was finished, Natasha came over and I introduced her to Nick.

"We goin' to Rumours next?" she asked me.

"Aye, let's go." I said as Nick was holding my waist. "Are you coming with us?" I asked him.

"I am indeed. If that's okay with yous, of course?" He looked at Natasha specifically then over to his mates. "You comin', lads? Rumours?"

"Fine by me." Natasha said, grinning as Nick's mates nodded and started following us.

Rumours was a nightclub about five minutes' walk away. Natasha was busy flirting with Nick's friends, while Nick and I walked together, him cuddling me with his left arm. It felt natural. As if I'd always meant to be there. Rumours was already busy when we arrived, it being a Saturday night, but we managed to get a space to stand and have a dance and a drink. The music was faster than at Brannigans, and tunes like 'Logical' by Scooter and DJ Otzi's 'Hey Baby' belted out whilst we all jumped about like idiots. Every now and then, Nick and I would look at each other and smile, or we'd stand together, him cuddling me from behind whilst I rested a hand on his. When the music stopped and the lights came on, Natasha came over.

"We off, then?"

"Two minutes, Nats." I turned to Nick. "Time for me to …"

"Can I have your number? I want to see you again, away from all this." "Yes! Me too!" I sounded a little too eager, but I didn't care. I read my number out and he sent me a message there and then. My heart fluttered a little as my phone beeped and I looked at the screen – Goodnight beautiful. See you v soon xxxx.

I looked up and smiled. "I have to go, Nick. She's away already." Natasha was just up ahead so I reached up on my tiptoes, breathed in Nick's aftershave once again and kissed him on the cheek. "Night Nick. See you soon."

I didn't look back as I hurried after Natasha, but I could feel him watching me go.

CHAPTER 8

After lots of texting and some long phone calls, Nick arrived at my house to take me on our first date, for dinner and drinks at a pub roughly equidistant between our two houses.

At twenty-eight, he was ten years older than me, recently divorced and living just outside of Blackpool with his parents. He had a young son whom he barely saw, and he worked as a phone salesman, driving round the north of England selling corporate phone contracts. I wasn't fazed by any of it: the age difference, broken marriage, even his son. Without having seen him in a few days, I'd grown fonder of him to the point I couldn't stop thinking about him. He was forever on my mind. I introduced Nick to Mum and Dad, and Dad did the usual 'friendly grilling', firing questions at him like "Do you drive?" "Where do you work?" and "You'll take care of her, won't you?"

Nick wasn't fazed by the questions, and he answered perfectly. "I drive, yes, but I'm safe," "I sell phone contracts, make good money too," and, "I'll look after Mhairi, she's a great young woman." Mum and Dad seemed impressed, and the tone was friendly, but nonetheless Nick and I were glad to leave to be on our own.

Nick turned to me and gave me a cuddle and a kiss on the cheek. "I've missed you so much since last Saturday."

"I've missed you too. Can't get you out of my head somehow," I giggled back.

He smiled and my heart melted.

When we sat down to dinner, Nick immediately took my hand, and we talked to each other as though we'd known one another our whole lives. We both liked eighties music, he'd been a footballer for my hometown's local team, coincidentally, and when I told him I'd been out celebrating my acceptance into nursing college he beamed with admiration.

"Ooh, so my girlfriend's a nurse-in-training, is she?" He smiled cheekily at me.

"Girlfriend? That was quick!" I said.

"It feels right though, don't you think? Will you be my girlfriend?" he asked.

"I think I could handle that, yeah," I grinned back.

We left the pub and Nick came to open the car door for me. He grabbed me by the waist and kissed me. Whatever I'd been feeling up to that point multiplied. Quickly. He was passionate and gentle and intense.

Things escalated quickly between Nick and me. When we weren't texting, we were speaking on the phone and we stayed at each other's houses regularly, becoming inseparable. We were electric together. We had a certain spark, the type you couldn't feign. We with each other all the time and when we were out, we'd hold hands and Nick would start dancing with me or wrap his arms around me for a kiss. If I had a day off from work, Nick would pick me up in the morning before his work and I'd spend the day sitting beside him with a map, being navigator for his day's appointments across the north of England. We'd have the eighties music on, singing along, and I'd work out how many contracts he needed to meet his targets. Nick's work started to get busier, so he'd often go away for a few days at a time, which was torturous for us both but before long it was September, and the time came where I started university and would be busy with my own work.

Nick would drive me to university and pick me up and I was so proud as I noticed other students eyeing him up. When I started to work in a local hospital near to his house, I'd stay there most nights, and he'd give me his key to let myself in and out if his parents weren't home. I still worked in the nursing home on my days off, and Nick would pop in and see me whilst I was working, and he quickly became a hit with the residents. He had a charm which ran through him that was irresistible. His cheeky smile would light up a room and he would have a laugh and a joke with the residents in the home.

By this time, my mum had started to work odd days here and there to help at the nursing home. She always worked the same area, close to Dad, which meant she looked after the same residents every time she was in. One lady in particular, Kath, became close to Mum. They shared a love of piano music and were often seen chatting away over a cup of tea. Kath was an old soul. She liked her cups of tea and used to play the piano before she became too ill, but she'd kept a lot of her old sheet music which was decades old and had frilly edges and tea stains on a lot of the pages.

Kath was one of the residents who had met Nick. One night, Mum was helping Kath to have a wash and get her nightdress on, before the drinks trolley came round with the nightly Horlicks and biscuits.

"I know that man, Joyce," she said to Mum one night. "I know him from before he met your Mhairi. He's married." When Mum finished her shift and came home, she told me what Kath had said to her.

"You can't be serious, Mum. There's no way he's married. He was married but they got divorced. Maybe she's just confused," I said.

"But Kath was adamant, Mhairi, that he was still married. Be careful. Please?" said Mum.

"I will. But I don't believe it," I replied.

Nick had been totally open with me. Showing me pictures of his first wedding, his son, telling me he'd been too young, and they'd drifted apart. When I saw him later, I asked him about it.

"One of the residents in the home says you're still married," I laughed.

"Aw bless," he replied. "She's probably thinking we're married and getting mixed up." He grinned his cheeky smile at me. "We'd be just as well getting married, you know. We act like we are anyway. Will you marry me?"

"Are you kidding me on, Nick? Don't mess me around like that," I replied.

"I'm not kidding. Will you marry me? I love you." I looked at him and saw he was serious. I was gobsmacked.

"Oh my god, yes! Yes, of course I'll marry you. I love you too." I started crying, my mind already racing ahead to what dress I would wear.

"Good. I better ask your dad though, eh? It's only right," Nick said.

"Yeah, I think you better. We'll stay quiet for now."

A couple of days later, I was working in the home and Nick came in. He waved at me and went into the office to see my dad. They were in there for about twenty minutes and my mind hadn't clicked as to what was going on. When they came out, my dad was beaming from ear to ear. Nick approached me slowly, pulled a small box out of his pocket and got down on one knee there and then.

"Your dad says it's absolutely fine, by the way. So, will you marry me?" He asked. Tears welled up in my eyes instantly as if it was the first time Nick had asked me the question.

"Yes, yes of course I will! Get up!" I gave him my left hand and he slid the shiny silver band on my wedding finger. A single diamond sparkled as I tilted my hand from side to side, admiring my engagement ring.

Nick got up and kissed me tenderly. Residents and colleagues were congratulating us, and it felt amazing. It was the happiest moment of my life. Everything was slotting into place for me. I had a good job, I was at university, I had a fiancé, and my relationship with my mum and dad was going well. To top it all off, Nick took me away to York for three nights to celebrate our engagement.

On our way back, we took a detour to the Trafford Centre in Manchester for some shopping.

"I need a new watch, so I thought we'd have a look in here," he said, as he parked the car.

"Nice. I'll help you choose."

"Better yet. I thought it might be nice to get us matching watches. Nice ones though. What do you think?"

"Oh my god. Really? Thank you. That'd be great. Where from?"

"Just round here." He nodded his head to a corner and then took me to the jewellers. There were so many watches in the window from little cheap everyday ones, right up to ones that ran into four figures. "I like these ones over here, look." He led me to some fancy watches that were just shy of £1,000 each. "They're gorgeous, aren't they? Would look good on you. A little addition to your ring."

"They are stunning, Nick. Pricey though."

"Don't you worry about that. Do you like any of them?" Slightly shocked, I scanned the display and pointed to a dainty silver watch, with a small, round, dark blue face. There were four stones. One at each quarter. Enough sparkle to indicate quality, but not too much to make it tacky.

"That one's beautiful. It's small enough for my wee wrists too. There's a bigger one next to it, Nick."

"Yeah, I like it too. Shall we get them?" I nodded and hugged him tight. We went into the shop and asked to try the watches on. They were beautiful and mine fitted on my wrist perfectly. "We'll take them please," Nick said to the assistant. "Is it okay if I do it on nought per cent though?" The assistant nodded and went to get the paperwork to fill in, while I just sat there ogling my beautiful new watch. I wasn't really paying attention to what was going on until Nick spoke to me.

"Problem with the finance. I don't know why. There shouldn't be. Maybe because I've been changing roles at work with going away so it's not set up properly yet?"

I didn't even question it. My heart was set on the watches. "I'll do it in my name then. You can just give me the money every month? Win-win."

"Are you sure? We can just leave it and I can just get a cheapy one."

"No, I'm sure. I'll do it."

It was the first bit of credit I'd applied for, and it went through first time. Why wouldn't it? I had a good job with good money and had never been overdrawn by so much as a penny. Twenty minutes later, we walked out of the shop with nearly £2,000 worth of watches on our wrist, and I had nearly £200 coming out my bank account every month for the next ten months.

CHAPTER 9

A couple of weeks later, Nick and I were in his car driving round his appointments. He was quieter than usual, and his caring, smiley expressions seemed muted.

"What's wrong?" I asked him.

"Nothing. It's fine."

"There's clearly something going on. You're too quiet. Tell me, Nick."

"I need money. Quick."

"Money? What for?"

"Child maintenance have come after me. I'm £1,200 behind and they're threatening me with jail. I don't know what to do. I can't leave you to go to jail, Mhairi. I couldn't live like that."

"Oh my god. What are you going to do? Can they really just send you to jail?"

"I don't have it and there's no way of me getting it. They can and they will."

"I don't have that kind of money lying about, Nick. I don't know how to help."

"Could you maybe get a credit card? I'd pay you back every month."

"I never thought of that. Yeah, I could try."

"Thank you. You're a life-saver!" And with that he was back to his usual loving, happy self.

Later that night at home, I sat down to apply for a credit card, and got one straight away. It would take a week or so until I had everything in place, but my limit was £2,500, so I had more than enough to help Nick. When the card came through, we drove to Liverpool, where he had an appointment to see his son, and where he would pay the money. I gave him my card and pin number and waited in the car for over an hour.

"You all done?" I asked when he came back.

"Yeah, all sorted thanks to you." He smiled warmly, and I just felt relieved I'd been able to help the love of my life out of a desperate situation.

Nick went away the next week for work down near London. He phoned me the day he was supposed to be coming home.

"I'm not coming back today. I've got car trouble. I think it's on its last legs. I'll try and get back tomorrow."

"Aw, that's not good. What's wrong with it?" I asked him.

"The garage said something about the suspension needing attention and the engine needing a lot of work. Might be cheaper getting another car. Fancy having a look when I get back? I've got appointments with work, but I know a garage we can go to when we're out."

"Yeah, no problem. I'll help you look," I replied.

"Also, is it okay to use the credit card to pay the bill? I don't get paid 'til next week. Sorry, I wouldn't ask but I just want to get home to you." Nick sounded sad and all I wanted to do was help him out and get him back home as quick as possible.

"Oh yeah, you've still got it anyway. Remember our watches come out next week too. First payment. We'll talk about it when you're home though."

"Thanks. Yeah, we'll sort it out." When he came back the next day, the car was fixed and the day after we were running about the countryside again, looking for his appointment addresses. The last one was early afternoon, so we went to the garage he'd told me about to look at used cars.

He went straight over to a gleaming white Renault Laguna that was only a couple of years old.

"Do you like it?" Nick asked me.

"I love it. It's big and will do you for ages. Are you going to go for it?"

"Yeah, I think so. Just need to sort the paperwork out."

We went inside and, after the usual sales patter from the salesman and the customary exchange of niceties, started to do the paperwork for the finance on the car. The details had to be phoned through, and about ten minutes passed before the sales guy came over to us.

"Everything okay, man?" Nick asked.

"It is and it isn't." He sat down at his desk. "The underwriters are happy to put the deal through, but they want a guarantor on the agreement as back-up."

"What's that?" I asked naively. Nick's expression was blank.

"Basically, they want another name on the finance deal in case of non-payment. It's their way of making sure they still get their money if Nick here doesn't pay," the salesman said.

"Oh well, that's silly. Of course I'll put my name on it. It's hardly likely he's going to do a runner with the car, ha-ha!"

"Are you sure, Mhairi? It's near enough four hundred quid a month!" Nick asked with a concerned look on his face.

"Yeah well, I'm not paying it, am I? If it gets you, us, the car then it's not a problem," I said.

"I love you. Thank you," Nick said.

"I love you too."

A couple of days later we went back to the garage, handed Nick's old car in, and drove away in his new car.

For a couple of weeks, things went smoothly. Nick was happy and I was happy. But one day, Nick picked me up in the car and he was in a foul mood.

"Get in," he barked as I opened the passenger door.

"All right, grumpy. What's the matter?"

"Nothing, just hurry up."

He screeched out of the street and turned the corner so quickly, I jerked to one side.

"Bloody hell, Nick! Slow down! What's wrong with you?"

"My work hasn't paid me. I've got no money until they do."

"Don't worry …"

"I've got bills! Bloody car, watches. I'm gonna lose the car." We were on the country roads now and he was driving round the bends like a rally driver causing me to jolt from side to side.

"Slow down, Nick!"

He ignored me and sped up instead.

"Nick please. You're scaring me. Slow down! Please!" I was shaking.

He kept ignoring me and kept driving too fast before slamming on the brakes at a junction.

"For god's sake, Nick! Don't do that again. It's just money! I'll pay everything this month to help you out. It's fine. You just need to talk to me, okay?"

His face settled slightly. "Do you mean it? Is that okay? I am so sorry I scared you! Are you hurt?" Nick's voice was calmer.

"No, I'm fine. Just drive. Nicely. It's okay. We're in this together. We'll get through it."

"Okay. I'm sorry. I just saw red for a minute. Forgive me?" He shot me a cheeky smile. "Please?"

"Yes. I forgive you. Idiot." I smiled back, still shaking.

Later that night I paid his bills for him, and a weight visibly lifted from his shoulders, and started looming over mine. But I was determined not to show it to Nick. He was going to Norfolk for the week for work, and I wanted our last night together to be enjoyable.

The week passed without incident, and Nick came back his usual smiley, happy self. We had a few good days before the mood turned sour again.

"I need to go to Liverpool to pay more money," he told me one morning.

"I thought that was all dealt with. You want me to come with you?" I asked.

"Yeah. It was. But now they want more money because my wages still haven't been sorted properly."

"You really need to speak to your work again."

"What the hell do you think I've been doing? I am trying to get it bloody fixed; you know?" He shouted at me.

"All right. Sorry! I know you are. They're just messing you around, that's all, and I don't have any more money I can spare, Nick. My card is maxed out and I can't afford anything else going out my bank every month."

"Oh, and I suppose that's my fault, is it?"

"No, I never said that. It's just I'm struggling a bit now and I really can't afford extras."

"Yeah. I get the message. See you later, Mhairi."

He got up and stormed out, without so much as a kiss or cuddle goodbye. His mood shook me a little and I couldn't get rid of this feeling that something was very wrong. He'd left his jacket lying on my bed and temptation overtook me. I looked in the pockets on the outside. Empty. I looked in the inside left pocket, next to his heart and pulled out a receipt. It was dated from his Norfolk trip, only it wasn't a receipt from somewhere in Norfolk. It was receipt from a Glasgow petrol station. I stared at the receipt a while before putting it back where I found it, tears streaming down my face with the realisation that the only reason there could be for him to lie to me was because he was cheating on me.

Then I remembered my mum's warning to me to be careful, and the resident in the home claiming he was still married. So, I said nothing. Instead, I waited until I next stayed at his house whilst working in the hospital. His mum and dad were out when I'd finished so, as usual, I let myself in with his key. I knew where his junk drawer was. The one where all the odd rubber bands, paperwork, unopened letters would go, until we'd tidy it out once in a blue moon. This was a big, deep drawer in his old oak chest of drawers in his bedroom. As I rifled through the papers, there didn't seem to be anything of interest: old phone bills, council tax, charities wanting regular donations. Then, a blank A4 brown envelope. I opened it, took the papers out and read the words 'Decree Nisi'. They were dated from May but far from being a signed copy of a completed divorce, they were blank in the space where Nick's name was meant to go. He wasn't divorced yet. I felt sick. Tears sprang to my eyes, and I started sobbing, holding the papers in my hand. I knew I couldn't just let this slide. I had to confront him.

CHAPTER 10

Friday night. Nick came home to his parents' house where I had been staying for work; I said nothing about the incomplete divorce papers that I'd found as I was still processing what I'd found out and trying to decide if our whole relationship had been a lie. It certainly seemed that way. Later that night, he drove me home and dropped me at the door.

"I won't come in, Mhairi. I can see you're tired, and I could do with an early night myself," Nick said as he parked outside my house.

"Okay." I replied. "I'll see you Sunday? Love you." I said it for the first time without really knowing if I meant it with all my heart. Normally I would have put up a fuss about him not coming in or not making the most of spending the weekend after he had been away all week together but this night, I was relieved to get back to my own bed and try to process what I'd found out. On the Sunday, around midday, Nick arrived whilst my mum and dad were out at work. He came in and came upstairs.

"Nick. Can you sit down? I need to talk to you," I said to him without my usual affectionate hugs and kisses.

"Oh, I don't like the sound of this. Am I in trouble?" he asked with a cheeky grin, sitting beside me on the bed.

"Nick, what's going on here? I know you were in Glasgow when you were supposed to be in Norfolk. I found a receipt in your jacket pocket after you left. And I know you're still married. Someone at the home recognised you and I'm ashamed to say, I looked through your stuff and found the unsigned divorce papers. This has all been a lie, hasn't it?" I stared down at my engagement ring, turned it round, and looked up at his face, to see it filling with a rage I'd never seen before.

"You crazy bitch! You did what? Why would you do that? We had a good thing here!" He was screaming at me, his face filling up with rage, as he stood up and towered over me.

"What do you mean had a good thing? Are you still married, Nick? Is she in Glasgow? And if she is, who is in Liverpool with your son, if he even exists?"

"Of course, he bloody exists. I kept meaning to tell you about my divorce but just never got round to it. And no, she is not in Glasgow. My fiancé is."

"I'm your fiancé though."

"No, my actual fiancé I live with. I don't wanna talk about this. I came over cause I need money. I need a grand. Quick."

"No! I don't have it. I told you. You've had everything I was able to get. And even if I did have something, there's no way I'd give you it now."

"I'm not leaving without something. I'll just take my DVDs back then and anything else I've bought, shall I? I'm not messing about, Mhairi."

"Nick, no! Don't do this! We can talk about this. Sort things out."

Tears started streaming down my face. I couldn't stop them falling one after the other forming a river down my cheeks. Nick was frantically taking DVDs off the big blue bookcase by the window. He was just grabbing whichever ones he could and was chucking them on the floor, one after the other. Suddenly, he rushed out of the room, then went downstairs. After a minute or two, he came back up with a roll of black bags, tearing one off and then started stuffing DVDs into it.

"Stop this, Nick. This is crazy!" I got up and went over to him holding my hand out and touching his shoulder, but he turned towards me quickly and shoved me so hard I fell back onto the bed. "Nick No! What are you doing? Please just stop!" There were two bags full of DVDs now, and I got up again to try again to get him to stop, even for a moment. "Nick! Please stop!" I screamed at him.

"Shut up. This is done. We are done," he said as he stooped to pick up the bags. I shot up and went towards the door. "Don't even think about it, Mhairi. I'm leaving. Don't try and stop me." Of course that was what I was going to do. I got to the door just before Nick and stood in front of him, blocking his exit. "Get out of my way. Don't be stupid," he said.

"No. I'm not moving." I didn't believe for one second that he would do anything to hurt me physically.

"Last warning. Move!" He was bright red in the face and his eyes were dark and stormy. I stayed where I was, defiant yet clinging to a tiny speck of hope that his red mist would clear, and we would talk things through. But he was too far gone. He dropped the two black bags he'd been holding and grabbed me by both shoulders. He swung me round quickly and shoved me. I felt my head smack the wall first and then a searing pain in my chest. I couldn't breathe properly no matter how much I tried to gasp a breath in. Coloured dots flashed back and forth across my eyes, and I looked up at Nick, in disbelief at what had just happened. His face was blank and vacant. The soft, caring man I had agreed to marry had disappeared. He went over to the bed and grabbed the big black and white fluffy blanket I kept folded up at the bottom. He tossed it onto me before turning his back on me to retrieve his bags. "Don't try and follow me. You best stay there for a while."

He picked up the black bags and walked out the door. I was still struggling for breath and still felt dizzy. And somehow, I was still managing to cry.

I sat against the wall for an hour. The dizziness subsided, and I caught my breath. But the crying didn't stop. No matter how hard I tried, tears streamed down my face. Even when I thought I'd stopped for a second, on came the next deluge. It got worse when my mum and dad came home from work. Silent rivers turned to noisy waterfalls, as I tried to explain to them what had happened. They hugged me and made me cups of tea whilst I told them everything that had been going on.

"Better you find out now than if you had actually married him," Mum said.

"What an absolute berk. He better not show his face here again," Dad quipped.

"I honestly don't think he will. It was all so final. There's no coming back from this at all. It's over. Just like that."

"You just concentrate on you, Mhairi. Plenty more fish in the sea," Mum said.

That didn't help. Even though I knew they were right, I didn't want another fish. I couldn't even contemplate another fish. But I believed it when I said it was final. Still the tears kept coming, and I took the next two days off sick from the hospital. I couldn't face going in. I was still spontaneously bursting into crying fits and my appetite had vanished. By the time I went back to work, I was managing to mostly control the tears, but I'd still have to excuse myself on multiple occasions to have a cry then wash the tears away.

About three weeks later I was just managing to hold it together enough to get through a whole shift without crying. I'd got home one day and had a letter waiting for me. It was from the credit card company. As soon as I saw it, I remembered Nick had never given me my card back. I opened the letter, dreading what I'd find. It informed me I'd reached the maximum limit, and my payments were being increased to cover them. I didn't understand why that would happen. There should still have been money left on it. Their office was closed so I couldn't even find out why.

I was on a late shift the next day, so I telephoned the credit card company in the morning. I asked how my card had reached its limit and they told me I had taken cash out of ATMs. I argued that I hadn't and the man on the other end of the phone assured me the transactions were real, citing three dates, one after the other. Then it dawned on me. It was Nick. He'd taken cash out of ATMs in the days following our break-up and maxed out the card. All in all, it was about £600. I tried to explain the situation again but ultimately it was my fault. The best they could do was cancel the 'missing' card and issue a new, yet useless one. When I hung up the phone, I saw red. I knew where Nick's dad worked so I telephoned him. He wouldn't come to the phone to talk to me, which left me wondering what Nick had said about our break-up.

Another couple of weeks went by, with me just holding on. I felt like a ghost just floating aimlessly from one place to another, not really existing but not really disappearing completely either. I'd sit for hours just staring into space listening to Faith Hill's 'There You'll Be' and Toni Braxton's 'Unbreak My Heart'. I didn't sleep much either, instead I took catnaps here and there, just enough to function. How could he do this to me, when all we ever seemed to have between us was love? I couldn't understand it at all. Christmas 2002 came and went and at the beginning of January 2003 I got a phone call.

"Is that Miss Hutt?" a male voice said.

"Yes. Who is this?" I replied.

"Hi. I'm calling because you're down as guarantor on a Renault Laguna that was purchased on finance last year."

"Yes, I remember the car. What's wrong?"

"There haven't been any payments made on the car for four months now and as guarantor you're our next point of contact."

"Look. I don't know where he is. He took my stuff; he took my money and he disappeared. I can't help you. Don't call again." I put the phone down then picked it up and left it off the hook.

It was the final straw for me. I was struggling to pay the credit card bills and the watches I had bought on finance. After I paid my digs to Mum and Dad, and my phone bill I barely had anything left. There was no way I was going to be landed with this too. It had been three months since I'd seen or heard from Nick, yet I was still paying the price of the break-up. The tears returned. I went to the kitchen and filled a pint glass with water then took it upstairs to my room. I had paracetamol in one of my drawers and got it out then sat in the spot where Nick had left me. I was in a daze of sorts. Knowing what I was going to do but feeling completely detached from it at the same time. I took the first two pills, then I took two more. I started thinking how easy it was. Just take some pills, go to sleep and you'll never know any different. I took another two in my hand and looked at them. Then I thought No! He's already killed me once. Not again. I couldn't let him win, so I put the pills in the bin and decided to stay alive and depressed instead.

CHAPTER 11

After that day with the phone call about the car, and the tablets, I decided Nick wasn't worth making my life a life that I didn't live. I loved him deeply. I invested my entire being in him and he was and always will be my first love. But I couldn't stagnate forever. The 2003 equivalent of Tinder was good old Microsoft Messenger and Yahoo chat rooms and that is where I went. I ended up speaking to a guy called Pete, who lived in Nantwich, about two hours away from me. We spoke to each other for a couple of weeks and then he invited me down to stay with him for the weekend. I took up his offer because what did I have to lose? It was never going to go anywhere. We were both young and single, but it was a classic rebound situation for me to get my confidence somewhere north of non-existent. Nevertheless, it was a fun weekend, and at the end I returned home, and we texted each other for about a week afterwards before it fizzled out completely. Some weeks passed, and I spoke to other guys online, but never met up with anyone else. One guy, Ian from Salford in Manchester, became a friend. We had swapped mobile numbers and texted each other every day to see how we were both doing. He knew of Nick, and he'd experienced a bad break-up the previous year too, so we had a mutual understanding and empathy for each other. It was the second week in March when I told him I was feeling unwell. He put it down to still being stressed over Nick, but I felt something was wrong. I'd been having stomach cramps the past few days not unlike my usual monthly cramps. I'd been feeling sick and just not right.

On March 13 I discovered why. I went into the bathroom with a crampy feeling and then a shearing pain shot through me, and I fell to the floor, suddenly sweaty and dizzy. I felt a warm, damp sensation between my legs and saw blood. I'd been due my period for a couple of weeks, but it wasn't so unusual to be early or late for me, so my initial reaction wasn't of worry or surprise, just of 'here we go again'. But when I managed to get up off the floor and take my soggy bottoms off, I saw a large mass in my pants. It wasn't your normal blood clots from periods, this was something bigger. As I looked at it, I was sure I could see some sort of baby formation. It looked like a baby but then again it couldn't possibly be a baby.

"Mum! Dad! Help!" I yelled from the bathroom. I heard them come up the stairs at some speed.

"What's the matter?" Dad asked.

"Look! Help me. What's this?" I asked. I started to panic and then to cry. I had no idea what was going on. Mum and Dad looked at the mass in my hands then looked sadly, but knowingly at each other.

"Mhairi. Were you pregnant?" Mum asked.

"What? No! Of course not."

"Mhairi, it looks like you were, and you've had a miscarriage, sweetie," Dad said.

I was stunned. How could I not know?

"Mum will help get you sorted, and we'll take you down to the doctor's, okay? Just to confirm what's happened."

I looked at them both. They looked at me with a little sadness in their eyes, as though they already felt the pain that I had not. Dad phoned the doctor's and was told to bring me down straight away with the suspected miscarriage. He had his arm around me in the waiting room and when we were called in by the doctor he sat next to me, gave the sample to the doctor, and put his arm around me again.

The doctor turned away and examined the sample then turned round with a sympathetic look in his eyes.

"I'm afraid you've had a miscarriage, Miss Hutt. From the looks of it, you were about eight weeks along. Is that about right?" I looked to Dad, then to the doctor and nodded slowly. From the first mention of the word 'miscarriage' I'd been hoping that it wasn't Nick's baby. It would have been more than I could have handled emotionally if it had been his. Now it was confirmed that it was Pete's from Nantwich. We hadn't had any contact since our weekend together. I hadn't even seen him on Messenger again.

"I'm going to phone the hospital and get a scan organised for you. The severity of your symptoms, falling to the floor with agonising cramps might mean an ectopic pregnancy and I want to make sure that what you've brought in is the complete foetus. If it's not, you'll likely need to go into hospital for a procedure to remove anything left behind. I'll give you some painkillers to take home with you for a few days."

"Okay. Thank you. Dad?" I looked up at Dad and started crying again as the realisation hit me that I had been carrying a tiny life inside me for the past couple of months. And now ... nothing. Gone.

Dad took me home and upstairs to my room. Mum was waiting and gave me a hug.

"Come on. Get changed and get yourself into bed. You need to rest until you go to hospital in case you bleed any more," she said. "I'll make you a cup of tea and you take your painkillers and try and get a rest."

"I'll let you know when the hospital phone me, okay?" Dad said.

"Thank you both," I forced a half-smile through tears.

Mum came up with the tea a few minutes later and helped me get into bed and get comfy. When she left, I looked at the painkillers at the side of my bed. For a split second I was tempted, once again, to take them all. They were stronger than paracetamol, surely I'd only need a few. There was more than enough there. But once again I pushed the urge away, took two tablets and curled up in the same position my baby had been nestling in in my now broken womb.

***

Three days later, Dad drove me to the hospital for a scan. I had to give a urine sample for a pregnancy test before I sat down. As I lay on the bed, still bleeding, the nurse squirted some jelly onto my stomach and rolled the scanner round slowly, whilst watching the screen.

"I can't see anything to indicate an ectopic pregnancy with the ultrasound. What I'm going to do is give you an internal scan, just to double check," the nurse said. She turned away from me on her stool and when she turned back, she had a massive, white wand in her hand that was about two inches thick and over a foot long.

"There's no way that's going inside me," I said. "It looks like it should be used on an elephant!" The nurse had a little giggle at me.

"At least you've still got a sense of humour. Don't worry it's just the top bit that goes in. The gel's cold though." As she was saying this, she was unwrapping a condom and rolling it down over the probe and lathering lubricant all over it. Then I had to lie there, legs apart while the nurse prodded and poked around inside with her wand. It seemed to take forever.

"It looks like you've had a complete miscarriage," she finally said. "Your uterus is empty. And your urine came back as negative. So that all points to you not being pregnant any more. Just rest up for a while because you're still bleeding quite a bit, but you should be okay."

"Thank you," I managed to squeak as I got dressed before leaving the room. On one hand I was relieved to not need to go into hospital. On the other hand, it really hit home that I had been pregnant; that, for a little while, I was going to have a child. My first scan should have been to check my baby was doing well and everything was progressing fine. Not this. My first scan shouldn't have been to tell me my womb was completely empty and I wasn't pregnant.

All of a sudden, a deep sadness hit me in my guts and in my heart. I'd lost my baby and it must have been all my fault. I'd been so stressed and upset, brooding over Nick that I hadn't even noticed the tiny changes that would have told me what was happening. I'd brushed off the metal taste of ham as a bad pack and just not eaten any more. I'd put my sore boobs down to pulled muscles from work. And my tiredness down to emotional exhaustion. But had I paid attention, I would have known and I could have saved my baby.

I stayed off work and uni for just over a week after that. When I returned there were lots of cuddles and sympathetic looks and comments. Everyone was lovely but there was a little piece of me missing now. My heart wasn't in it any more. I told Ian what had happened and he suggested a break away together. I jumped at the chance. A week in the sun with a friend who knew me well enough to be comfortable around but not well enough that I'd be worrying about judgement. So, we booked a week in Crete in early April. Mum and Dad thought it was a great idea for me to get away.

"Just be careful, Mhairi," Dad said. "Look after yourself and enjoy it."

"You'll feel much better after a wee break in the sun," Mum said. "Have a fantastic time, and just forget everything here."

It was parental advice I was glad to take.

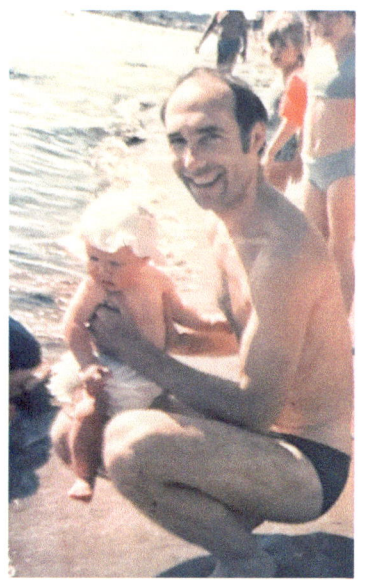
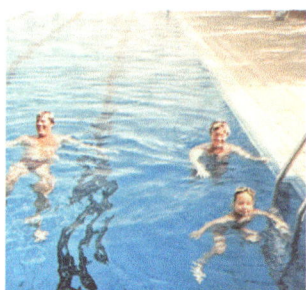

Top left: My first introduction to the beach with my dad. Largo beach, Fife, 1984. Top right: Swimming with family friends. Jeddah, 1987/'88

Below: Our apartment complex. Jeddah, 1987/'88

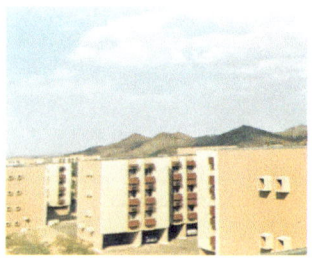

Right: Mum and I in our apartment. Jeddah, 1987/'88.

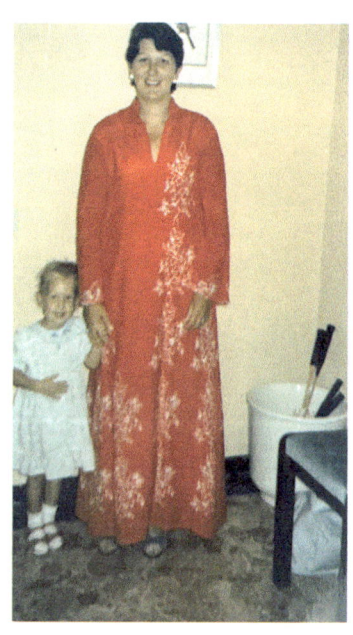

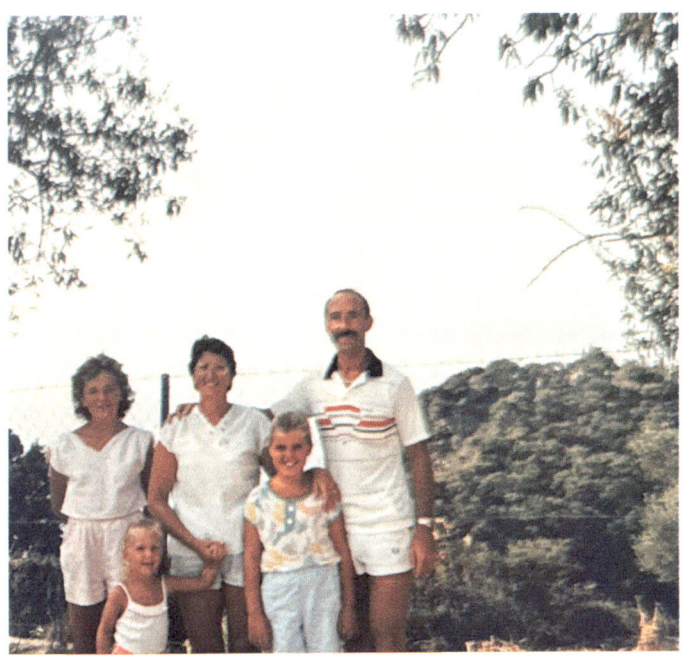

Top: A rare holiday when the five of us were together. Unknown, 1988

Bottom: Enjoying a happy moment with my older sisters, Lesley (middle) and Sharon (back). Kirkcaldy, Fife, 17th September 1989.

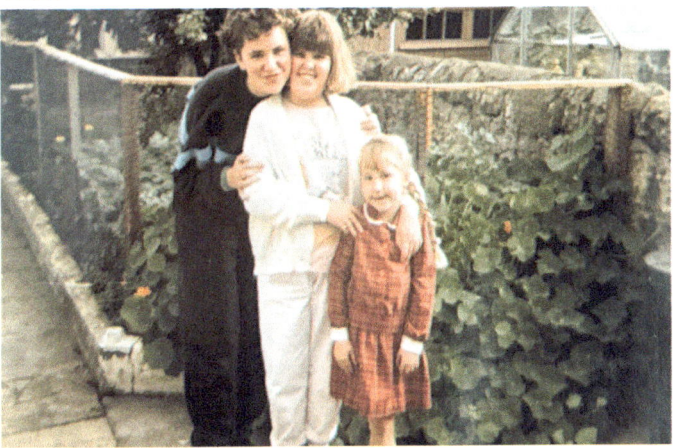

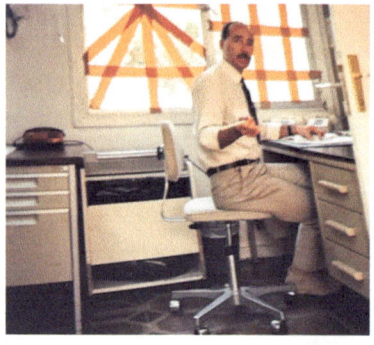

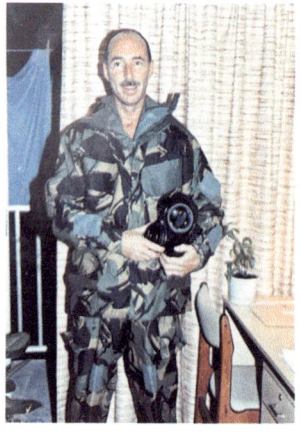

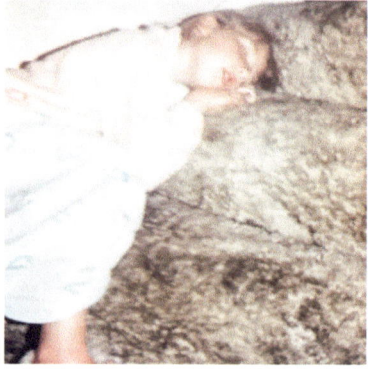

Above: One of the times I fell asleep on the stairs listening to Mum on the phone to Dad. Kirkcaldy, Fife, 1990-'92.

Below: Nana and Papa on their golden wedding anniversary. Kirkcaldy, Fife, 1995

Top left: Dad at his clinic in Saudi Arabia during the Gulf War. He had to tape the windows up to prevent them being blown in by bomb blasts. Dhahran, 1990.

Top right: Dad in his camouflage suit holding his gas mask. Even non-military personnel were issued with these in case of chemical attacks. Dhahran, December 1990.

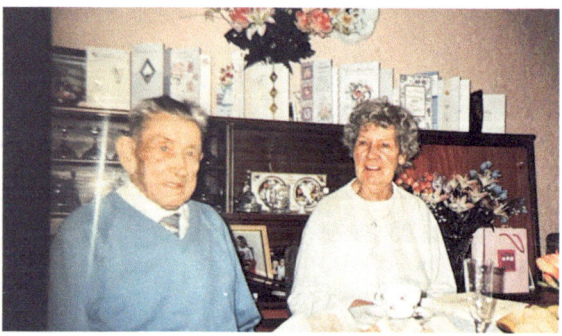

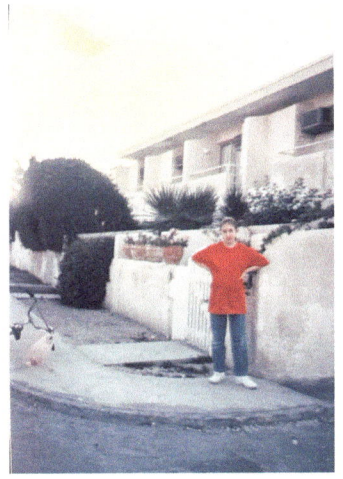 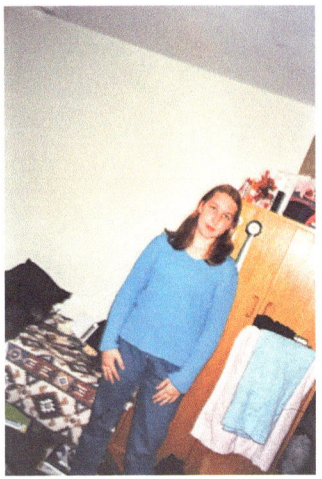

Top left: Outside my villa on Al Rowdha compound. Dhahran, 1996. Top right: Me in my dormitory at boarding school. Kirkham, Lancashire, 1997.

Below: The caravan Mum and Dad purchased for when they visited me at boarding school. Kirkham, Lancashire, 1996.

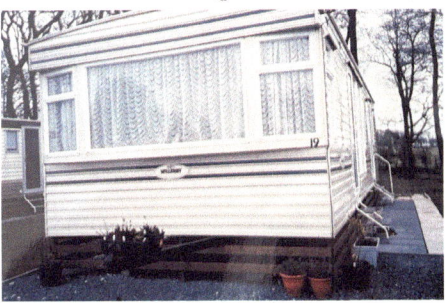

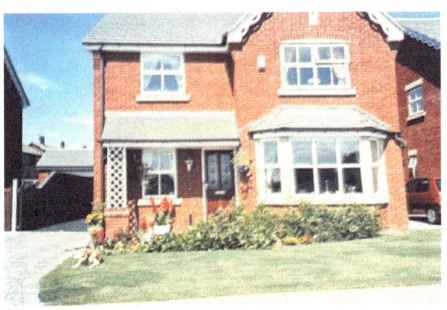

Left: The house we moved to when Mum and Dad left Saudi Arabia and I became a day pupil at school. Elswick, Lancashire, 1999.

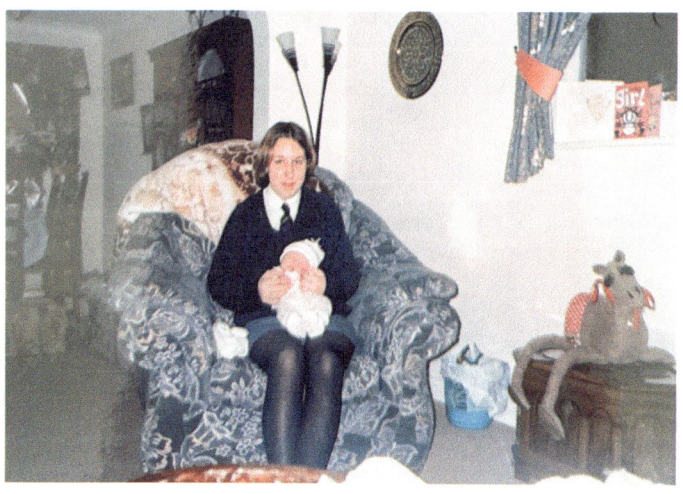

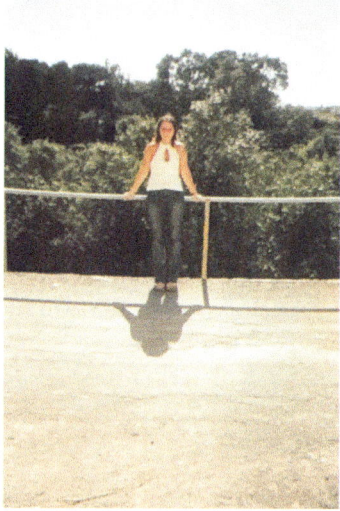

Top: Me with my newborn niece, Cerys. Elswick, Lancashire, 2000

Left: In Crete after splitting up with Nick and leaving nursing college. Hersonissos, 2003.

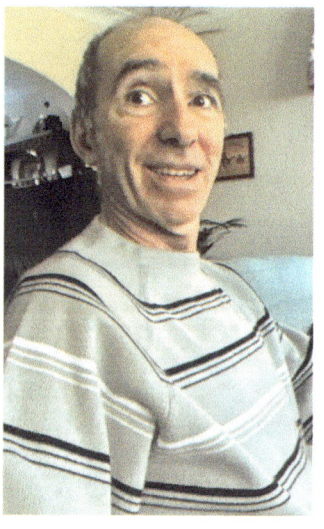

Right: Dad, after his brain haemorrhage, visiting home. Elswick, Lancashire, 2006.

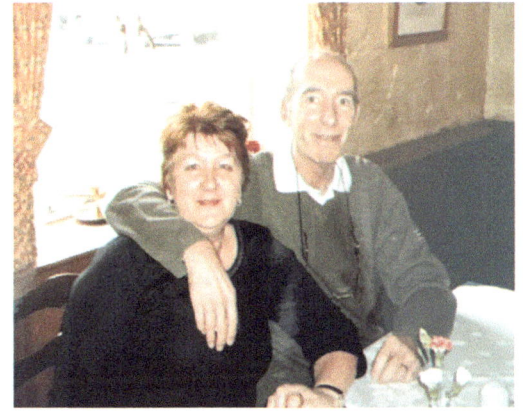

Left: Mum and Dad back together again. Lancashire, 2006.

Right: The house we bought in Inverness needed work to make it safe for Dad. Highlands, 2006.

Bottom: Gary and I on our wedding day. Gretna Green, 16th September 2015.

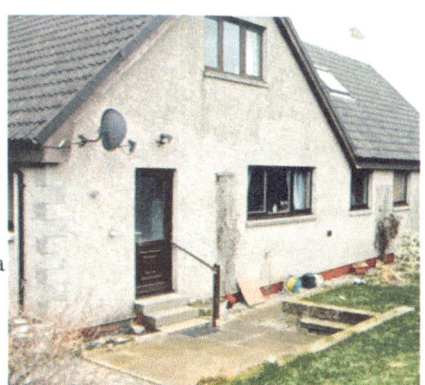

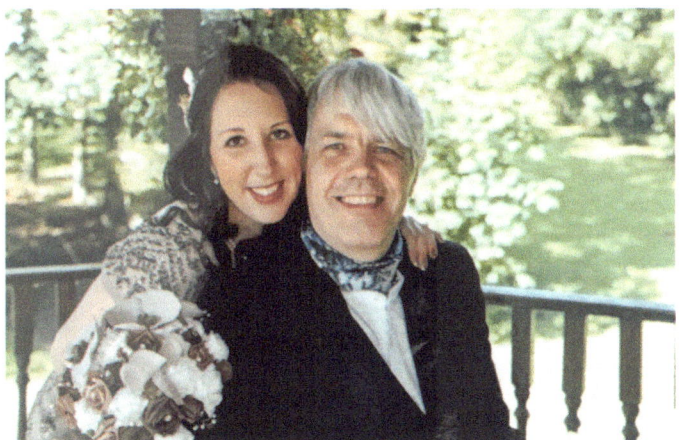

CHAPTER 12

Ian and I stayed in Gouves, a little village just outside Hersonissos in Crete. Although our relationship was platonic, we were sharing a room, which was slightly on the awkward side of comfortable. There wasn't much to do in the hotel, so we went into Hersonissos every day to explore, often walking up and down the beach road and harbour. It was hot and peaceful and every moment I was there I felt the stress of the break-up with Nick and the acute heartache of losing my baby slowly slip to the back of my mind.

I fell in love again. Not with Ian, but with Crete, the culture, and the feeling I had while I was there. Nobody knew me, nobody had any preconceptions of who I was, and, more importantly, nobody had any expectations of me either. I felt the healing process had begun, and by the time the week was over, I was sad to be leaving my little haven.

When I arrived back home, I immediately felt unsettled again. The sensation of dread returned. I felt once again the urge to disappear from life, and I decided within a couple of days that I couldn't remain at home like this. I called the university and told them everything and asked to defer my nursing course for a year. They agreed and wished me well, telling me I'd hear from them in September. The hard part was telling my parents.

"What are you doing that for?" Dad asked. "You've just started your nursing at university. Don't throw it away like this."

"I'm sorry, Dad, but I feel like I need to do this. The past year has been horrible for me, and my heart is no longer here. I can't be here and look at everything the same way as before. I need to go away and sort myself out. To be free of everything. I hope you can understand, even if you don't approve."

"I understand, Mhairi," Mum said. "You're hurting and you need time away. It's okay. You go back to Crete. Just promise you'll stay in touch and stay safe."

"Thank you. I will, I promise." I got straight onto the computer and booked a one-way ticket to Heraklion airport for £80. There was no point in booking a return. I didn't know when, or if, I was coming back. I booked a nice hotel in Hersonissos for four nights. I figured that was enough time to find my own apartment, and more importantly find a job.

I boarded the plane nervously, not knowing what lay ahead. Four hours later, my nerves still hadn't subsided. If anything, they'd gotten worse, and I began to wonder if I was making a mistake. After collecting my bags and getting a taxi to take me the twenty-five-minute ride to the hotel, my stomach was gurgling, and I felt sick. As soon as I got into my hotel room, I went to the bathroom and vomited, shortly followed by explosive diarrhoea. After that, I immediately felt better. I took a quick shower, changed into a long, white, floaty skirt, an off-the-shoulder black crop top, and black flip-flops, before making my way down to the beach road and a few of the bars I was familiar with. Some of the bar staff recognised me and welcomed me back, surprised to see me so soon. One barman from Romania, Steven, was especially pleased to see me, and over the next couple of days he helped me to find an apartment and a job by acting as a translator. He helped negotiate with the elderly Greek lady who owned a six-apartment block, for a first-floor apartment for €300 a month.

My new olive-green apartment was small, but quite comfortable. It had a small, mosaic-tiled bathroom, with a toilet, sink and shower. The only other room was a kitchen area with a sink, double-ring cooker, two cupboards on the bottom, and another two above. A single wardrobe stood opposite the bathroom, and a wood-framed double bed occupied the largest space. I had my own balcony overlooking the street to the right and the beautiful blue Sea of Crete to the left. It was stunning and I loved it.

I got a job in an Indian restaurant which was owned by a couple from London and managed by their two sons. The hours were 5pm until the last customer left, often around midnight, and sometimes as late as 2am. I worked hard to pay my rent, but I partied hard too. My days began around 11am or noon, when I'd shower, eat, then sunbathe. After work, I'd be straight out to the bars and clubs, often until 5 or 6am. Many sunrises were spent walking the quarter mile up the rough beach path from the club strip back to my apartment. I got friendly with quite a few of the locals, and I'd spend time drinking raki with them and trying to improve my Greek. I was living the good life, and I got to the point that I allowed myself to be a little bit happy for the first time in a long while.

I'd taken my engagement ring with me to Crete. I didn't know why I'd taken it, but at the beginning of my stay I'd sometimes look at it and remind myself of Nick and our time together. I wore it occasionally, but never on the finger where it used to belong.

One morning, as I was heading to the beach, I picked it up. I kept it in my hand as I walked the fifty metres to the beach, but instead of going to lie on the sand, I walked up the rocky outcrop and stood on the edge, looking out to sea. I realised that the ring meant nothing to me any more. With a final glance, I threw it as far as I could into the waves below. Maybe some archaeologist will find it someday; maybe somebody already has. That same day, I went to a boutique that stocked Greek designer dresses and shoes. I bought myself a pair of six-inch stiletto heels that criss-crossed halfway up my calf, and I also treated myself to a strappy, layered dress in shades of brown and gold that had frills round the hems. That night, I went to a local Greek club and partied until dawn in my new outfit. I felt free.

About a month into my stay in Crete, I became friends with my next-door neighbour from Belgium, Lakshmi, and my neighbour directly above me, Nikos, from southern Crete. Lakshmi, like me, was here to escape for the summer, and Nikos worked every summer in Hersonissos to earn extra money for his parents who owned an olive farm. Nikos used to bring me two litres of retsina and a litre of olive oil whenever he'd been back to his parents' farm. Lakshmi and I spent many a night out together and we'd often go to Malia for the day to go to the beach. It was packed, but there was good music and always some sort of party going on.

One day, I left the beach on my own to get back for work. It was only a ten-minute walk from the shore to the main road where I could get the bus. On the way, I stumbled across a Scottish bar. I say stumbled because I was happily hammered in the mid-afternoon sun. My boss never minded, just as long as the work got done. It was just how it was. I went into the bar to get some water and to my surprise, the owners were from Kirkcaldy. The walls were littered with football shirts, scarves, and pictures of Raith Rovers football club. On the wall, there was a team photo from the 1992/93 season. I remembered my first date with Nick. When I'd mentioned I was from Kirkcaldy, he told me he'd played for Raith Rovers that season. I studied the photo for a minute or two and realised, unsurprisingly, that he wasn't there. I had a little silent chuckle to myself the rest of the walk up to the bus stop.

***

While I was in Crete, Michael started texting me out of the blue. I hadn't heard from him since I stayed in my flat with Sarah in Kirkcaldy back in 2001, but my memories of the time I spent with him were fond ones, so I replied, and we rekindled our friendship via long-distance texts. I filled him in on my life over the past year, and he was understanding and caring. He told me he would never treat me like that, and that Nick had no idea what he'd lost. It got to the point where I would get a little fluttery when I saw Michael's name pop up on my screen.

In July 2003, I told Michael I was coming home. My periods were getting to the point where I'd be crippled over in pain for two or three days at a time, so I just needed to be at home. Michael was delighted and promised to phone me as soon as I was back home. I flew back home and made an appointment with the doctor, who suspected I had picked up an STI. A few days later, I got the results: I had chlamydia and needed antibiotics. I was absolutely mortified. I'd been sensible enough to take the pill whilst I was away, but not sensible or sober enough to use condoms. My infrequent school attendance had caught up with me in my total lack of sexual health awareness. Ashamed of my naivety, I told Mum and Dad I had a urine infection, and when Michael did at last phone me, I told him the same story.

Within a week, I felt better. Despite nightly calls from Michael, and my relationship with my parents improving, I decided I wasn't finished with Crete. In the second week of August, I flew back out to resume my restorative summer. This time, I was so worried that I would catch something that I decided sex was off-limits for the remainder of my time there. Before I left, Michael had said he'd wait for me to come home. We'd grown close and had all but declared our love for each other, so in my mind I wasn't single any more. Michael wasn't at all like my usual type. Nick had been my type. Michael was 5' 9", skinny, with a shaven head. He wasn't your classic good-looker, but his tenderness, protectiveness and his wicked sense of humour had won me over, so I was willing to give things a shot.

I lasted in Crete until mid-September before I decided I'd had enough, and it was time to go home for good at last. Mum and Dad were pleased, though I got the feeling they didn't believe I was going to stay for long. They both questioned whether I was ready to come back, and kept asking what my plans were, and had I thought things through?

Michael was happy. He couldn't wait to come down from Kirkcaldy to Elswick to visit me. I was just as excited. He came down for a few days in October, and we decided we wanted to be with each other during that time. He was so kind and caring, and we stayed up for hours just talking about everything and nothing. When he went home, we both promised it wouldn't be long before we'd see each other again and that we would make our relationship work over the 230 miles that separated us.

Over Christmas and the New Year, Michael and I spoke every day, even if it was just for a minute or two. He worked days as a fabricator, and I was back on shifts in the nursing home. I'd missed starting university for that year, which meant I'd forfeited my place and would need to decide if I wanted to restart my entire nursing course the following year. I'd already decided I wasn't going to do it, but I hadn't told Mum and Dad yet. The time for studying had come and gone, and the very thought of reliving that time made me sick to my stomach. In January 2004, the distance separating me and Michael was too great, and we decided we needed to be closer. Michael offered to move down to Elswick, an offer I gladly accepted. I was happier at home than I would have been up in Kirkcaldy. I just had to clear it with Mum and Dad.

"Are you sure about this?" Dad asked. "He's more than welcome to come here, but we are just worried about you.

So long as he pulls his weight, he can come. Joyce, what do you think?" he asked, turning to Mum.

"I agree. We just want you to be happy, and if this is what you want, then fine. Like your dad says, so long as he if he helps then he can come down."

"Thank you so much! He will!"

It was as simple as that. Michael was down within a fortnight. He couldn't find work as a fabricator near where we lived, so he came to work in the nursing home with me and Dad. It was hard because we rarely worked the same shifts as each other, but most weeks we managed to get a day off together. It made it easier that he got on well with Mum and Dad too. Things were so good that by early March, Michael had asked me to marry him. We were just sitting in my bedroom one day, when Michael turned to me.

"Mhairi, I don't have much to offer you. We're not rich and I can't really afford a big shiny diamond, but I know I love you and I know you love me. Will you marry me?"

"Oh! Well, I wasn't expecting that. I don't care about money, Michael. Yes, I'll marry you. I don't care about a ring either. I'd wear a plastic one if that's all we could afford."

We went one better than a plastic one – we spent £25 at the jewellery section of a local supermarket on a silver-plated ring with cubic zirconia stones round the band. I didn't bother about the price tag because for the first time since Nick, I could see a life for me with somebody else, with Michael. Mum and Dad were happy for us too, but sadly it was overshadowed just a week later. Michael phoned his parents back in Fife. I watched him pacing around the garden, talking on the phone, his brow furrowed. His cheeks started to redden, and his eyes started glistening. When he eventually hung up, he sat down on the patio and put his face in his hands. I hurried outside.

"What's wrong, honey?" I asked, as I sat beside him and cuddled him.

"It's my dad, Mhairi. He's dying."

He broke down completely, sobbing into my lap and I couldn't help but cry with him. William was his idol, and a kind, generous soul. He'd been a racing driver, and had even won some big Scottish races in the past. Michael was eager to follow in his footsteps, and they often went to races together, bonding over fixing up old bangers into race-worthy contenders. I knew this was a devastating blow for Michael.

"Oh, Michael. What's happened?" I asked.

"He's got liver cancer. It's too advanced to do anything. He's only got a couple of months left."

"Oh god. I'm so sorry, Michael. Do you want to go up and see him? I can come with you."

"I think I need to. But I think I need to go up to stay until he … until …" He broke down again, returning to my lap.

"Okay. Well, that's what we'll do. We'll go up and we'll look after him. I'm quite able to do it, and between you, me and your mum, we'll make sure he's comfortable and can stay at home. How does that sound?"

"Are you sure? It means leaving here again, and I know you didn't want to go back to Fife."

"I'm sure. I'll sort everything with my parents, and we'll go as soon as we can."

"Thank you. Thank you so much."

Within a week, we had packed up our stuff and made the three-hour journey up the road to Fife. We stayed in Michael's parents' house, in Michael's old room. William looked so thin and frail compared to the healthy, strong man we'd seen only a couple of months previously. Within a couple of weeks, he was completely bedbound. Michael, his mum and I took turns washing and caring for William. He was still conscious, but the liver cancer ravaged his body, turning his skin an orangey-yellow. He was on a morphine syringe driver – an electronic pump attached to a syringe which automatically administered morphine to him – which made him sleep most of the time.

One afternoon in April, I was helping William to get comfortable. He was lucid, more lucid than he had been in some days. As I helped him to take a drink, he held my hand and looked at me.

"You'll look after Michael for me, won't you? When I'm gone?"

I paused for a moment, taken aback by his directness and by his acceptance of his impending death. I'd seen many people die when working in the nursing home, but nobody had ever been so blunt. Most of the residents who'd passed away were in their eighties and nineties, and generally went into a comatose state for a couple of days, before gently passing away with one of the nurses or family by their side. This was different. William knew his time was coming, and it was as though he needed to tie up his loose ends before he finally let the cancer take him.

I looked into his eyes. "Of course I will. For as long as he wants me to. Don't you worry about that. You just concentrate on you, William." I gave him a tearful smile and a gentle cuddle.

Later that night, Michael and I were woken up by a loud knock on the bedroom door.

"Michael! Mhairi! It's Dad. He's asking for you, Mhairi. Come down."

"Just coming," Michael replied. He went to get out of bed, and I held his arm.

"Michael. Be prepared, okay?"

He nodded knowingly, and we both went downstairs where William was sitting up in bed. He gave us a weak nod as we came in.

"Mha ... iri ..." he pointed his finger up. He was fading away before my eyes.

"You want me to help you up the bed a bit?"

He gave a half nod in reply. I looked at Michael, then at his mum, who smiled through her tears. I sat down on the bed beside William and put my arms round him, gently pulling him forward while Michael readjusted the pillows and added a couple more to sit William up a bit. When I lowered William back onto the pillow, the relief on his face was clear to see. He blinked his eyes, gave a little smile, and lay his head back, holding my hand. I looked up at his face and his eyes were closed. A little trickle of blood fell from his nose, just touching his top lip. I watched his chest slowly rise then fall, slow and long. After a minute or two, I realised his chest would not rise again. I stroked his hand a final time. I looked up at Michael, and then his mum. Now I had tears in my eyes.

"I think we should call for the doctor. He's away."

CHAPTER 13

Michael and I stayed with his mum for a month after William died. We then decided it was time to get our own place together. We wanted to stay in Fife to be near Michael's mum. I got a job in a nursing home in Kirkcaldy, just fifteen minutes away. Some of Michael's friends were working for a local scaffolding company, and there was a job there for him when he was ready to start.

I found a flat for us three miles away from Michael's mum in East Wemyss, an old coal mining town. The furnished flat was on the ground floor of a building that used to be the local pub. It would cost us £395 a month, but for that we had a sun lounge, large living room/kitchen, two double bedrooms and a bathroom. There was even a back garden that the six flats in the building shared. The décor was tired, with chipped magnolia paint and green-and-cream striped wallpaper that was peeling off at the corners and yellowed from the nicotine stains of previous tenants. The dark blue sofas dipped in the centre, so when you sat down your knees were higher than your hips. The beds wobbled and creaked, and the ageing peach bathroom suite had black mould growing in all the corners. It was a start at least, and we were glad to have our own space. The stress of the past few months had taken its toll. My periods were erratic and heavy, bringing migraines on a weekly basis. I was put on Pizotifen tablets for the migraines, which made me sleepy, and the doctor suggested I could have ovarian cysts which were contributing to the bad periods.

Michael wasn't coping well after his dad's death. He started drinking every night once we moved into the flat. His mood changed, we'd have regular shouting matches when he was drunk. I was reminded of Nick, and I tried to hold onto the hope that this would pass with time, and we would get to a better place soon.

On September 4, I woke up to a wet bed. I lifted back the covers to see blood. I sat up, and felt a searing pain shoot through my abdomen. I called the doctor, and they arranged an ambulance to take me to the hospital, as Michael was at work. On the way, I called him, and he said he'd meet me there. The paramedics gave me painkillers because I was writhing about so much. I was given a bed in A&E, and soon afterwards a nurse came round with a scanner. As she was setting up, I felt a familiar wet, warm sensation, and I began to weep as I pulled back the sheet. I knew what had happened. It was just like my first miscarriage. The nurse turned to me and gave me hug.

"Ah, you poor thing. Come here. I'm so sorry." She said to me.

She held me for a minute while I calmed down.

"Do you still have to scan me?" I asked,

It was a rhetorical question; I knew she would.

"I'm afraid so. I need to check if everything has come away or if there's still something there. And check for an ectopic pregnancy. I'm so sorry. I'll be as gentle as I can and as quick as I can. I'm going to need to get the doctor in here to look at you too, okay?"

I nodded through my tears. I had to wait half an hour for the doctor. He examined my stomach, examined the mass I'd passed, and stood watching the screen as the nurse scanned me. I watched the screen through tears, as the nurse moved the scanner firmly but with care over my now empty belly. The doctor turned to me.

"Your uterus doesn't seem to have anything there that would suggest you need any further treatment. By the look of what you've passed, you were seven, maybe eight weeks pregnant. I think if you're okay, you can go home. Just make sure to get plenty of bed rest for the next four or five days. If you're still bleeding heavily after that, or if you pass any big clots or have a lot of pain, then phone your GP. I'll make sure you get painkillers to go home with. Does that sound okay? I'm so sorry. Is someone coming for you?"

"Yes, thank you. My fiancé is coming to get me. He doesn't even know. We didn't know I was pregnant. Just like the last time, I had no idea."

"The last time?" the doctor asked, raising his eyebrows.

"Yeah, I had the same thing last year. I didn't know I was pregnant until this same thing happened."

"Okay. Please rest up for a few days. If this happens again, we might need to get you in for further investigations. The nurse will help you clean up a little"

"Okay. Thank you." I turned to the nurse. "And thank you too."

"I'm so sorry again, Mhairi. I'll get some wipes for so you can freshen up a bit, and I'll get a pad for you to put on until you get home."

Michael came in about ten minutes later. I burst out crying.

"What's wrong? What's happened, Mhairi?" He hurried over to me and wrapped his arms around me.

"I've had a miscarriage, Michael. I didn't even know I was pregnant. I'm so sorry!"

"Shhh. It's not your fault, darling. Don't worry. We'll get through this. We just need to get you home and get you some rest, okay?"

"Okay," I cried.

We went home, and for the first couple of days, Michael was off work and took care of me. He made sure I stayed in bed or on the couch with my feet up. He was so attentive and brought me cups of tea and helped me get dressed through the pain. I was grateful because with my first miscarriage, even though Mum and Dad looked after me, it wasn't the same as having somebody you love, the father of your baby, help you and go through the grief with you. He barely left my side those first two days. After that, he went back to work and when he was home, he was slightly less attentive. I put it down to grief. It hadn't been long since his dad had died and now, we'd lost a baby. It was a lot to take in at once. So I wasn't altogether surprised when he began having a couple of beers at night when he got home from work.

After a week, I began feeling better and went back to work, and often joined Michael in having a drink to relax at night after a hard day. Things went back to normal for a while. We even got a little black-and-white kitten, whom we named Squeak. She was a cheeky wee cat, running up and down the curtains, and hiding under the beds. By the time Christmas came round, we were trying to stop her hiding in the Christmas tree and playing with the tinsel. It never stopped her though. She was sweet when she wanted to be. She'd often curl up on the sofa beside me when Michael went to the pub after work, which tended to be at least three times a week. He'd stay home the other nights, but never without stopping off at the shop to get some beer for the evening.

Four months later, in January, I was doing a fourteen-hour shift at work in the nursing home. Just after lunchtime, I was helping take one of the residents into the lounge for the afternoon. I felt a horrible pain punch through my stomach, without warning. I fell to the floor with the intensity of the pain and pure shock. I started sweating, went cold, then felt a wave of nausea come over me. It being a nursing home, the place was of course full of nurses and care assistants, and the duty nurse was called straight away. She managed, with the aid of another carer, to help me to the toilet, just in time for me to vomit and have diarrhoea. The next thing I knew, there was blood in the toilet.

"I need the hospital," I managed to say to the nurse.

"I think that goes without saying, Mhairi. The ambulance is already on the way."

"Thank you. Michael?"

"We'll call him for you and get him to meet you there. Don't worry. We'll get you sorted. Just sit there and wait for the ambulance, okay? I'll get you cleaned up a bit and get you some fresh clothes."

I nodded and looked down at my vomit-covered tunic and the mess I'd made on the floor. I was so embarrassed. I just wanted the ground to swallow me up. But I knew the pain. I knew the signs now and it was confirmed when I got to the hospital. It was different nurses and doctors, but the process was the same. I got painkillers and I was scanned to check if there was any of my third baby left inside me. There wasn't. Again, I was roughly eight weeks pregnant, and had had no idea. Michael arrived shortly after the scan.

"You didn't know at all? How?" he asked, quite unsympathetically.

"I don't know. It was like last time. I didn't feel anything. My periods weren't as heavy but everything else was the same. I didn't notice anything."

"Surely there was something?" he pressed.

"No! There was nothing, Michael. Can we just go home? I need my bed."

He nodded and helped me out to the car. When we got home, he made sure I had everything I needed, then he went back to work. There was no looking after me this time. It was unsettling.

For the next few days, I barely saw him, except when he would get home, stinking of beer from the pub, or briefly in the morning before he left for work. I knew he was grieving, as I was, but I couldn't help feeling that we should be sticking together. I didn't have the strength to bring it up, though. It was like it was me that was the problem; it was my fault I had lost the baby, so I felt I had no right to question how he was dealing with things. I just hoped things would get better.

Instead, things with Michael were getting steadily worse. One day, we were driving home from getting a grocery shop and were three miles from home when Michael pulled over to the side of the road.

"I can't help thinking you did something," he said.

"Did something? What do you mean?"

"The baby. You had to know you were pregnant. How could you not know?"

"I didn't, Michael! I had no idea I was pregnant. Do you not think I already blame myself every single day for losing our baby? If I'd known I was pregnant, I would have stopped smoking. I would have started taking vitamins. I would have done anything and everything, but I didn't know."

"Get out! I don't believe you. Just get out of the car. You can fucking walk home."

"What? No! Why are you being like this? Michael?"

"Get out of my fucking car. Now!"

I got out. I didn't know what else to do. I didn't want to make him any angrier than he was. He was suffering too. I shut the car door and watched tearfully as he screeched away down the road and left me standing there. I waited for about twenty minutes, sitting on a nearby bench, hoping he'd have a change of heart and come back for me. But he didn't.

I walked home. When I got in, he didn't speak to me, and I didn't speak to him. I didn't know what to say, so I just put the shopping away and we spent the rest of the day in complete silence. When we spoke to each other the next day it was like nothing had happened. He was completely fine and didn't mention anything. I thought it safer to act the same. There was no sense in provoking him.

Michael's drinking started to get more frequent. Within a month of my losing the baby, his drinking had got so bad that he lost his job. One night, he didn't come home after work. This wasn't unusual in itself, but by midnight I was beginning to worry. His phone was going straight to voicemail. I sent texts, asking if he was okay. I didn't hear anything until he came in the next morning, looking the worse for wear, and smelling of stale beer.

"Where have you been? I've been so worried about you!" I went to give him a hug, but he shoved me away. It was the first time he'd laid his hands on me with anything other than affection.

"Get off. I'm not in the mood."

"Not in the mood? I've been up half the night wondering if you were okay. What's going on?"

"Got stopped by the police doing sixty in a thirty. Drunk."

"Oh, Michael!! What did you do that for? You could have just got a taxi home!"

"Well, too late now. Got court in a couple of days. Probably just get a fine, though."

"Well, let's hope so."

A few days later, after his court appearance, he came home with a £300 fine, and a twelve-month ban from driving. He also became jobless after having phoned his boss to let him know the bad news about his driving ban. His licence was a must for his job. So, with no licence he had no job. Michael was furious. Furious at his boss. Furious at the court. Furious at me. He went to the fridge and got a can out, popped it open and sank into the couch. I tried to talk to him.

"Look, it was a silly thing to do. But we'll manage okay. You can get another job and we'll manage fine without a car. It's never as bad as it seems. I'm starting my new job next week, so I'll be able to pay the fine until you get back on your feet." I walked over from the kitchen area to the sofa and sat beside him.

"You think? Just leave me alone. I'm not in the mood." He shot me a filthy look, so I got up and left him to it. He fixed his stare on the floor, taking frequent gulps of beer. It wasn't even lunchtime. By teatime he had gone through eight cans. He'd only moved to get up to go to the toilet or the fridge. He'd not said a word to me the whole time.

"Do you want some dinner? You're bound to be hungry by now."

"Why? Cos I'm drinking? What else should I do?" He had an angry glint in his eye.

"I'm just making some dinner and wondered if you wanted some. You've not eaten all day and, yes, if you must know, because all you've done is ignore me and drink and I think some food might do you good."

My patience was wearing thin now. I could take a lot but, in my mind, he was being nasty to me for the sake of it.

"No wonder I've been drinking." He got up from the sofa, and walked towards me. "Lost my job. Lost my car. You lost my baby. Lost my dad."

"It's not like I meant to lose the baby, Michael. I didn't even know I was pregnant. Both times. I had no idea. I'm sorry. I've apologised so many times. I am sorry though. I don't know what else I can say! You can't blame me more than I blame myself."

I was crying by now. I didn't know how he could be so cruel. He walked right up to me and pressed his nose right up against mine, pinning me to the kitchen worktop, staring straight into my eyes.

"You better be sorry. It's your fault I'm in this mess. Not mine. Get it?"

He spoke calmly and pointedly, not raising his voice but I could feel the anger pouring out from him. He nudged my head with his and turned away from me. He swung his arm back and turned slightly, then punched the wall full force, knocking a hole right through the plasterboard. I let out a scream and he turned without looking at me and went through to the bedroom, slamming the door behind him. It was a tearful dinner for one that night.

After that night, things were quiet for a little while. I started working at a newly opened DIY shop and started making some friends. I never finished later than 8pm, so the hours were good and allowed for some social time in the pub afterwards, and the odd dinner out for workmates' birthdays. Michael was still jobless, but he'd slightly cut down on his drinking. Nevertheless, things weren't the same as they had been before he punched a hole in the wall. The hole, which had never been fixed, served as a warning to tread carefully.

"My work's looking for folk in the garden centre if you're interested," I said to Michael cautiously one night.

"Really? Do you think I should apply?"

"Yeah, I think you should. It's only part-time, but it would give us some extra cash. Everyone's nice and you'd make pals there too. I brought a form home with me in case you wanted to fill it in." I was surprised at how well he was reacting to me even suggesting he get work.

"Okay. Give it here. I'll fill it in and hand it in tomorrow. I'll come in on the bus with you when you start."

"Cool. I've already put a good word in, so you never know."

"Thanks, Mhairi."

"No bother."

He was as good as his word. He filled the form in and took it down to the shop the next day when I started my shift. He got an interview the day after that and, within a week, he'd started work. As I did, he really liked the job, and got on well with everyone. We rarely worked together, as Michael was part-time, and I was full-time. This meant he was often at home while I was at work. But I found myself working as hard at home as I did at work. I'd come home to piles of dishes, packets, and cans on the floor and on top of the unmade bed. The washing would pile up until I had a day off to start doing it and the cat litter tray would be left unscooped and stinking of cat wee.

"Michael, would it be too much to ask if you could just tidy up after yourself? I'm not asking you to scrub the house from floor to ceiling, but if you could just put your rubbish in the bin and scoop Squeak's litter tray, that would be a massive help to me."

"Are you joking?" A little flicker of rage crossed his eyes as he looked straight at me.

"No, I'm not joking. I'm just asking if you could do those couple of things to help a bit, that's all. I'm working forty hours a week. I'd appreciate a wee hand." That was the wrong thing to say.

"Oh, and I suppose little Michael doing twenty hours doesn't mean much, does it? It's not my fucking job!"

"I'm sorry, what? It's not your job? Michael, I'm not some little wifey who's going to stay in the kitchen. We've always been equal, haven't we? I can't do it all."

"Well maybe you should reduce your hours and I can increase mine. Then the house will be tidy!"

"What? Don't be stupid. I like my job. I'm not cutting my hours so you don't have to pick up after yourself. That's ridiculous."

"So now I'm stupid?"

"No, you're not stupid. I said don't be stupid. The idea is stupid, not you!"

Michael got up, went over to the bookshelf under the window, loaded with books. He grabbed it with both hands and toppled it over.

"Your books. Your mess. You clean it up."

He walked out of the house.

I was so angry, but also a little shaken. It was like a red mist had enveloped him and he couldn't see through it. I pulled the bookcase up off the floor and sat down to restack my books. I felt that I was the problem. It was my fault I'd lost our babies, so this was the least I deserved.

CHAPTER 14

The situation continued to worsen. I'd come home from work to find the house in a mess, and just clean it up, not saying anything to Michael that would aggravate him. He'd started drinking again, and the flat often smelled like stale beer from the empty cans lying around. I knew the signs to look out for by this time. If the smell hit me when I came in from work then I'd just quietly go about my business, cleaning up and making dinner. If he was staring at the floor, I wouldn't bother clearing up around him, I'd just busy myself elsewhere. He was often drunk going into work, but he hid it well with extra doses of mouthwash, chewing gum and aftershave. We barely spoke at work, and I was lucky if two pleasant words were exchanged between us at home.

"Are you okay, Mhairi?" Simon asked me at work one day. Simon worked full-time like I did, and we'd been out on various works nights out. He was a little taller than me at 5'8". He had hazel eyes and short, brown spiky hair, with bleached blond tips. He was eighteen months younger than me, but he seemed mature for his age. He had a slender, toned frame and a chiselled jawline. I'd never really spoken to him much, just occasional pleasantries at the pub or in passing at work.

"Yeah, I'm fine, ta. Just a little tired. I'll work it off though."

"Okay. But if you need to talk about anything, I'm good at listening. Look, take my number just in case, okay?" He handed me a piece of receipt paper with his number on it. I took it and put it in my pocket.

"Thanks. I'm fine though."

But I knew that he knew I wasn't. He sometimes worked with Michael, and I'd seen them talking together a few times. I didn't know what he might have been told by Michael, but it must have been something for him to show an interest so suddenly. Nevertheless, I put his number in my phone and texted, Hi, it's Mhairi. Thanks for today, later that night. He replied, No problem, and that was the end of it.

I didn't give Simon another thought until a few weeks later when there was a works night out coming up. It was on a Sunday, which meant the shop would shut at six so that whoever wanted to go could do so. Some of us took clothes to work to get changed into, while those who lived close to work, like Michael and I, went back home to change. Then we all met up in the bar and started drinking and dancing and having a good time. At about 10pm, Michael came over to me. I hadn't seen him a lot during the night. We'd been socialising with other people.

"Time to go home," he slurred.

"What? I'm not going home, Michael. It's still early and I'm having fun."

"You're coming home now!"

"No, I'm not! You go if you want but I want to stay. I'll not be too late."

"Oh, I get it. You want to stay out without me so you can have a good time when I'm not here, eh? Well, that's not going to happen." He grabbed my arm and dragged me outside the pub.

"Let go!" I screamed. "You're hurting me, let me go!"

Simon had followed us outside.

"Let her go, Michael. You can't be doing that. Just leave her alone."

"You get to fuck. Want her, do you? Here, you can have her. She's no' worth anything anyway." He shoved me towards Simon but luckily, he was so drunk it didn't have the same force as him dragging me outside. I stayed on my feet.

"Shut up, Michael. You're acting crazy," I yelled. "Just, let's both go home, okay? We'll get a taxi and go home."

"Do what you want." He was already walking away.

Simon gave me a look, as if to say, don't go with him, please. I gave him a silent apology and hurried after Michael, knowing that to stay would be a dangerous mistake. Michael had told me to stay, but he didn't mean it. When we arrived home, silence ensued once again, but Michael was so angry that he punched two more holes in the walls, one in the hall and one in the spare bedroom, which was where he slept that night.

The atmosphere wasn't any better the next day, and it only worsened when Michael went to the shop and came back with a case of beer. He didn't even bother putting it in the fridge; he just sat on the sofa, staring at the floor with the open case beside him. Over the course of the day, the case emptied, as the floor filled with discarded cans. I stayed in the bedroom as much as I could, only coming out for food, drinks, and the bathroom. Simon had messaged me to check if I was okay, and although I hadn't told him how bad I thought things were, he seemed concerned enough to tell me to get out of the house and meet him in town, so I didn't have to sit at home with a drunken Michael. I couldn't, though. Me leaving the house then would have been tantamount to taunting him. He wouldn't have let me leave. I was stuck.

It was teatime before Michael said anything to me at all. He came into the bedroom.

"You making me some tea?" he said.

"Okay. What do you want?"

"There's bacon and sausage there. Just use the grilling machine," he said, almost ordering me.

At least you're talking to me, I thought, as I got off the bed. I was trying my hardest to stay away from anything I thought might set him off into a rage, so I just did as I was told. I made dinner and gave it to him. We sat and ate in silence. When we'd finished, I took our plates and put them on the worktop next to the grill.

"I'm just going to get stuff ready for work tomorrow, then I'll clean up, okay?"

There was no reply. I waited a few seconds.

"Michael?"

Still no reply, so I left the room and went to the bedroom. I'd only been gone fifteen minutes when I went back through the kitchen and found Michael standing at the worktop, looking at the dishes and the grill.

"You no' cleaning this mess up?" Michael asked.

"Yeah, I said to you before that I was just going to sort work stuff for tomorrow then I'd clean the dishes up."

"That's not fucking good enough!!" He yelled right up in my face. He looked mean. Angrier than I'd ever seen him before. He unplugged the grill, took it in one hand and grabbed me in the other. He marched through the living room, into the sun lounge and out the front door, with me shouting "Michael!" and "Stop!" every couple of steps. He threw the grill onto the road and pushed me after it. I cowered.

"Now you'll clean up your mess," he sneered and turned around, going back in the house and slamming the door behind him. I stood there, in the middle of the road, crying uncontrollably until I heard the beep of a car horn, and turned to see it racing towards me. I jumped out of the road and watched as the grill got bashed about the road in the car's wake. I went back onto the road and picked up the mess. Cradling the grill, I walked back through the front door and into the sun lounge. I stopped momentarily. It was silent. I walked through the sun lounge into the living room, feeling a whoosh of air brush past my cheek. I stopped and looked at the floor, as I heard a thud on the carpet. The breadknife I'd used not an hour before was lying at my feet, having narrowly missed my face. I looked up at Michael in complete astonishment.

"Did you just throw a knife at me? What for? This is crazy, Michael! Please stop this now! I don't know what I've done to deserve this. Please stop and tell me how I can make this better."

"You can't make this better. I'm just sorry I missed."

He was in a rage. He picked up the cat's scratching post and threw it at the kitchen door. The door was glass-paned, and three of the panes shattered at the impact.

"Michael, stop!" He stepped over the glass and disappeared into the spare bedroom. I was still standing at the doorway to the living room holding the broken grill. When Michael left the room, I quickly went over to the kitchen and put it straight in the bin. I retrieved the knife and stuck it in the sink then went through to the spare room, dodging the broken glass. "Michael, can we talk about this? I understand you're angry at me. Please can we try to fix this?"

He looked up, with a menacing smile.

"You think we can fix this? You think you can be fixed?" he snarled. He backed me up against the wall. With his left hand, he held my neck, and with his right hand he made a fist, which he pushed into my cheek.

I was shaking. I thought, He's going to kill me. He meant to hit me with that knife. He's going to strangle me instead.

He was right up in my face now. "You don't know how much I want to hit you right now."

He's not going to kill me. Think, Mhairi. Think.

"It would be so easy to do it, you know. But you're not worth doing the time for."

From somewhere deep within, I found my voice. "You know, if you want to hurt me, you can punch me in the kidneys. Right there," I whispered, unable to speak any louder over his hand closing round my throat. I pointed to my right kidney then took his fist and placed it where I'd pointed. "Just here. It would hurt me. Probably give me internal bleeding. But nobody would see it."

His eyes cleared, and he looked at me properly for the first time in days. He let go of my throat and backed away.

I felt a surge of bravery. "Go on, Michael. Hit me! Right here!" I pointed again. "That's what you want, isn't it? To hurt me? Well, do it, you fucking coward!"

He stared at me and said nothing.

"No? That's the last time you make me feel like that. No more. Do you hear me?"

He said nothing, so I left the room and went into the bedroom, shaking. I needed to shower and change my clothes. I realised I'd wet myself with fear.

The next morning, I awoke to find Michael sitting on the sofa. He was staring at the carpet. I expected to see empty beer cans beside him. But there were none. He was just sitting, staring at the floor. In the past, I would have just ignored him, got on with my day and quietly avoided him until he spoke to me. But I was tired of being a victim. The grill in the road, the bread knife, the strangling, it was all too much, and any fire that I had suppressed within me came erupting out. Whether it was right or wrong, what followed was the only way I knew how to hit back at him and get him away from me. It was either this, or one day I truly believed he might kill me.

I messaged Simon. I'm going to kick him out. I've had enough. Last night he took it too far. I'll text you when he's gone. I knew Simon had been worried when I'd been dragged away from our night out, and I wanted someone to know what was going on in case I needed help.

"What are you doing, Michael? Don't pretend that you're the victim after last night. Are you even sorry for what you did? For what you were going to do?"

He said nothing.

"Not talkative this morning? Maybe this will get your attention!" I went over to my bookcase, the one he'd upended not that long before, and I tipped it over. The thud of it hitting the floor made him jump, but still he sat silent. He didn't even look up. On the windowsill there were three model racing cars that Michael's dad had built. "Maybe this will wake you up!" I grabbed the first one and threw it on the floor, watching as it smashed, bits of plastic flying across the room. I picked up the next one.

"What are you doing, you fucking psycho? Stop it! They were my dad's!"

"At least now I have your attention."

I picked up the next car and threw it down next to the first. More shattered plastic flew across the room as Michael stood up and came towards me.

"No way," I said with a completely calm, emotionless voice. "Don't even think about coming any closer or I'll throw this one too."

He stopped, rage flickering in his eyes. I could tell all he wanted to do was hurt me, grab me, and exert some sort of threat over me.

"You can have this back, but first you'll listen. I'm sorry you lost your dad, Michael. But that was over a year ago and at some point, you have to start moving on. You need help with that. You're a drunk and I'm not to blame for that. Losing the two babies wasn't my fault, and as much as I want to blame you for it like you do me, I won't. Nobody knows what causes them to be miscarried and I won't let you make me feel responsible either."

He was stared at me.

I was still and calm. "I want you to go. Take what you can and get the f*** out of this flat. What you did last night will never happen again. I hate you with every inch of my body. There's a bus due in twenty minutes. I suggest you get on it. I'll send the rest of your stuff in a taxi when I can be bothered. You'll get this car as you're leaving. Okay?"

He nodded and turned to go through to the bedroom. I kept hold of the car and went to the dish on the worktop where we chucked our keys at night and removed his house keys. I wasn't leaving anything to chance. I stood and waited until Michael came back through with a blue sports bag and a black bag full of his belongings.

"I've got some stuff. Can I have the car?" he mumbled.

"No, not yet. You can have it when you're outside. I'm not stupid. I've taken your flat keys. I'll phone up tomorrow and get your name off the list. Oh, and I'll stop paying your fine too. Time for you to go." I nodded towards the door, and he started walking. I followed a safe distance behind him just in case he decided to do anything stupid at the last minute. He opened the door and went out. I put his keys in the door and made sure I had a grip on the handle.

"Car?" he mumbled again.

"Oh yeah, sure. Go fetch, you absolute bastard," I replied as I lobbed the model car into the road, hitting almost the same place that the grill had landed the night before. He watched as the car smashed on impact, then turned around to come at me, as I slammed the door and locked it in his face. He was shouting and screaming through the letterbox, hammering on the windows for a good half an hour before I finally saw him standing quietly at the bus stop. I watched him get on, then burst into tears, releasing all the fear I'd built up whilst making sure he left. I was so relieved.

I messaged Simon. He's gone! His reply was instant. I'm coming over. In case he comes back. Simon came over and stayed to make sure I was okay, and to be there if Michael came back. He didn't, and the only time I heard from him was to chase me up to give him his stuff, which I took over a week to send to him via a taxi. I still hate portable grills and I won't use them.

CHAPTER 15

Simon never really went home. He stayed with me for the first few nights after I'd thrown Michael out, just in case he came back, but after that he stayed because we'd grown close, shared a few kisses, and one thing inevitably led to another.

But I was guarded. My break-up with Nick, three miscarriages, and Michael had left me feeling distrustful and sceptical that nothing good was going to come of Simon and I giving a romantic relationship a try. Nonetheless, I let it play out. He was kind to me, and deeply caring. He helped around the flat, making sure that he tidied up after himself and never let me do more than my fair share of the chores. It was a refreshing change.

When he did go back home, he texted or called me frequently to make sure I was okay and, when I had my fourth miscarriage, he couldn't have been more supportive. Like the other three, I had no idea I was pregnant. I just had bad cramps one afternoon, and then the familiar blood and tissue came away from my womb. I didn't feel the need to go to the hospital, instead I phoned the doctor and went down to be seen. The doctor examined what had come away and confirmed that it looked as though I'd been eight or nine weeks pregnant this time – the furthest any of my pregnancies had got. The doctor didn't feel the need to send me to hospital, as I knew what to look out for if anything untoward was happening. Instead, he gave me the now familiar painkillers and advice, and told me to "carry on as normal", "think about going back on the pill" and "try again for another baby – it'll do you good." Flummoxed about how trying for another baby would somehow do me good, I left the doctor and phoned Simon.

"I've had a miscarriage, Simon. I'm okay, just a bit sore and sad. I'm going to go home and get some rest. I'll phone work and tell them I won't be in for a few days."

"I'm here at work anyway. I'll tell the boss and let him know you'll phone in later today or tomorrow. You don't need to be worrying about that today. Was it ...?"

"Yeah, it was Michael's. I can't imagine how that conversation would go if I'd had to let him know I was having his baby. It's weird, I'm not as upset about this one. Maybe a blessing in disguise."

"But still, you can't be feeling great about it. I'll come over after work and see how you're doing, okay?"

"Okay. Thank you."

True to his word, Simon came over after work and made sure I was keeping my feet up and not doing anything.

We spent all our free time together. We'd sometimes have friends round to the flat for parties, where we'd all get too drunk and regret it the next day, especially when some of us had work. Michael still worked at the same place, but he never came on nights out any more, and I acted as if he didn't exist at work. Nobody knew what had happened, though I suspected he'd spoken to a couple of people, giving them his side of the story, because there was a definite rift in what had previously been a unified team. Some people started to avoid and ignore me, and some would avoid and ignore Michael. For the most part, it was still a nice place to work. I hadn't told Mum and Dad about the full extent of our problems, nor the final break-up. I spoke to them every couple of weeks or so just to catch up on events. It was usually Mum that phoned me, or I would phone, and she'd pick up. So I was surprised to answer the phone to hear Dad's voice one day. Even more so, when I realised that he was calling me in floods of tears, and couldn't get his words out. I immediately thought something was wrong with Mum.

"Dad? Dad, what's wrong? Is it Mum?" I'd never heard my dad cry in my whole life. There'd never even been any hint that he was capable of it, and yet here he was sobbing down the phone.

"Topsy. Ma wee Topsy's died. What am I going to do?" he wailed.

"Topsy? The cat? Oh, thank God! Well, no, not thank God. I thought Mum had died! Oh Dad, I'm so sorry. She was such a lovely cat. Glen will be sad. He'll be missing his cuddle with her."

"What am I going to do? Ma wee Topsy, Mhairi. My poor wee Topsy."

"It's okay, Dad. I'm sure she's in a better place now. Aw, I wish I could give you a cuddle. It'll be okay."

"Okay. Here's Mum."

And that was it. Topsy, our cat from Saudi Arabia, had died, and Dad was beside himself with grief. It was like he was mourning the loss of our whole lives in Saudi Arabia. Like a part of our lives was now dead and buried. It broke my heart to hear my dad cry like that.

The next time I heard from my parents, I was in Dumbarton. I'd been offered the opportunity, along with a few others at work, to go from Fife down to Dumbarton to conduct a stocktake of that store. I jumped at the chance. It was two days away with workmates, no customers, and having a bit of a drink and a laugh at night. We got there in the afternoon, and got straight to work emptying shelves, cleaning them, counting the stock then putting everything back. It was tedious, but a change from our usual routine in the store back in Fife. At night, we had a meal at the hotel then sat in various rooms drinking, which must have gone on into the wee hours, as I don't recall getting much sleep. In the morning, with heavy heads, we made our way to breakfast, before a full day of counting screws and nails began. I was just finishing my fry up when one of the managers, Jim, came over to the table.

"Mhairi. You need to call your mum. She's just been on the phone to the shop looking for you. Something about your dad."

"My dad? Okay, I better go. Thanks, Jim." I got up, went outside, lit a cigarette and dialled home.

"Hello?"

"Mum? Jim's just told me to phone. Is everything okay?"

"Oh, Mhairi. Your dad's not right. He's been in the hospital. He collapsed at work. His BP was sky-high. Something like 210 over 120. They sent him home though. Said it was a bad viral headache."

"Should he not still be in the hospital?"

"Well, I think so, but they said he'll be fine. He's got painkillers and he's in bed, but he doesn't seem well at all. He was being sick and was really confused."

"I'm coming down. I need to see for myself. I'll get down as quick as I can, okay? Message me to keep me updated. It'll be okay, Mum. He'll be fine."

"Okay. I'm worried, Mhairi."

"Just hold on. I'll be there as soon as. I'll let you know what train I'm on. Love you. Tell Dad I love him too, will you?"

Something wasn't right at all. Dad was a fit and healthy fifty-eight-year-old. He'd been working at the home and collapsed while doing his rounds that morning. The staff had managed to get him onto a bed, then called an ambulance, and called Mum. When he'd got to the hospital, he'd had his basic observations done at the accident and emergency unit, and he'd been diagnosed with a viral headache, given paracetamol, and told to go home to sleep it off. I was more than worried. I was terrified he was going to die. A blood pressure reading that high was a sure indicator a stroke was happening. There was no way he should have been at home. I let my bosses know what was happening, and they told me to go straight away. I packed my bag and got the train from Dumbarton down to Preston, where Mum picked me up to drop me at the house, before heading to work to sort some things out.

I arrived at the house, and went straight upstairs to see Dad. It was awful. He was lying in bed with his eyes wide open, not in a good way like they normally were though. His eyes were scared, searching for something. They were flitting from side to side, and up and down.

"Dad? It's Mhairi. Hi."

It took everything I had not to burst into tears. He heard me, and about five seconds later, he finally saw me. He mumbled incoherently, before stretching his arm out of the covers and opening his hand to reach for me. I stepped forward and took it, sitting on the bed next to him. I fell onto him, giving him a massive hug.

"Aw, Dad! I don't think you're very well, are you?"

He looked at me and shook his head. He could barely focus on me, couldn't speak, and just kept trying to touch my arm. He looked like a lost child, completely alone, with no idea what was happening. I decided to phone our doctor's surgery rather than an ambulance. The receptionist put it through as an urgent call and the doctor came out within the hour. When he came up to see Dad, he looked at him, then looked at me, and I knew he was thinking the same thing I was.

"Ooh, that's rather high, Allan," he smiled at Dad, as he finished taking his blood pressure. "I don't think you should be at home. I know you're not long back from the hospital, but I think you need to go in again. I'll phone them for you though. Is that okay?"

Dad blinked in agreement. He didn't even have the energy to nod his head any more.

The doctor came over to me. "I can't believe they let him out! He should not be here."

"I know. That's what I thought. Thank you for coming out. The sooner he's back in hospital, the better. He's not very well at all, is he?"

"No, he's really not a well man at all. You did the right thing. I'll go and phone the ambulance."

"Thank you. I'll go and let my mum know."

I looked over to Dad. "The ambulance will be here soon, Dad. I'm just going to phone Mum."

The ambulance arrived and took Dad to hospital, while Mum met us there. Dad was put on the medical admissions unit and hooked up to all sorts of machinery. He was drifting in and out, with moments where he looked more lucid. Once he'd settled in, Mum and I visited him, before going home for the night. The nurses assured us that he would be looked after. They'd see what tests he needed, and they'd call if anything happened or they had news. I was worried, and reluctant to leave Dad alone in the hospital, but I knew he was in the best place. They'd look after him. They'd get to the bottom of what was wrong with him, and he'd be on the mend in no time, back to his usual cheeky, fiery self.

The next morning, we hadn't heard anything. Mum decided to call the ward to see how Dad was doing. She sat at the desk in the study while I clung to the doorframe, waiting for news. But there was a problem.

"What do you mean you don't know who that is? He was only brought in yesterday ... The name's Hutt, yes. Well, I suggest you find out, because nobody has told us anything." She put her hand over the mouthpiece and looked at me. "They don't know where he is!"

"What do you mean they don't know where he is?"

"He's not on that ward. He's been moved. She's just away to see where to."

"For goodness' sake!"

Mum turned her head back to the phone. "Yes? Okay. What's the number? Thank you." She hung up. "They've found where he is. He was moved in the middle of the night. That's all she said. I'll try this number now."

"You want a cup of tea? Kettle's just boiled?"

Mum nodded as she dialled the new number. By the time I got back with the tea, Mum was looking concerned. She had a pen and notepad, and was scribbling furiously. She wrote something down and pushed the paper over. Arrested twice. Haemorrhage. Might not make it. I looked at her in disbelief, standing there with two cups of tea as the news sank in. Mum finished the call. I put the tea down and hugged her.

"He's had a massive bleed on the brain. Not just one but two. Subarachnoid haemorrhage, the nurse said. It was so big they had to resuscitate him twice. They didn't think he would come back, but he did. Now, against the odds he's clinging on. But he is clinging by a thread. He's unconscious and has had seizures. They said we better go in just in case it happens again, and he doesn't come through. Someone should have phoned us."

"I can't believe they didn't! I'll be having a word with someone when we go in. That's not good that nobody thought to tell us he'd moved wards for a start. Or that he's died twice!"

I was numb going to the hospital. Neither Mum nor I could quite believe what we'd been told. We knew he was ill, but nothing prepared us for hearing we'd nearly lost him, had lost him twice. We shouldn't have been surprised that he pulled through really. He was super-fit for his age, helped by his five-day-a-week tennis hobby in Saudi. He was strong-willed, determined and a force to be reckoned with when he had to be. He had to be now. He had to pull through. There was no way he'd just give up. By rights, the bleeds should have killed him. But that wasn't the worst of it. It should never have got so bad. If the hospital had scanned his brain and given him a lumbar puncture when he was first admitted, his bleed could have been, at best, prevented, or, at worst, insignificant. His blood pressure alone should have alerted the hospital to a bleed on the brain. But they ignored the signs and told him he had a headache, so now he was in critical condition.

CHAPTER 16

When Mum and I arrived at the hospital, it was worse than anything I could have imagined. I'd worked in nursing homes and in hospitals, but nothing prepares you for seeing your dad in the same position you've seen so many patients in before. He was a shadow of a man, even more so than when I'd seen him in his bed the previous day. He was unconscious, and hooked up to the vital signs monitor which measured his pulse and blood pressure. I could see he was catheterised too. His face was covered by an oxygen mask, helping him to breathe. He had an ECG machine next to him, beeping away, and I could see he had a central line in, too. The cot sides on the hospital bed had been raised and covered with padding in case he started fitting again.

His pale, lifeless body lay there, still, unaware that we had even entered the room. Mum went straight over and held his hand. I went to his medical notes at the bottom of his bed to get a better picture. After the hospital had failed to contact us, I didn't feel I could trust what they had told Mum over the phone. Sure enough, flicking through the notes, I stopped at catastrophic bleed and GCS 5. Seeing it in black and white made me shiver. The bleed should have killed him, but instead he was effectively comatose. The Glasgow Coma Scale runs from three to fifteen, with three being akin to being brain-dead, and fifteen being fully awake, aware and able to function.

"Mum? This doesn't look good at all. His GCS is only five."

She turned round and I saw her tearful face. "He's strong, Mhairi. He'll fight and come back to us." She turned back to Dad and leant down. "Won't you, Allan? You listen to me now, okay? You fight and come back to us. Don't you keep us hanging on. If you're coming back, you stay and fight and you come back. Do you hear me, Allan?" She looked back to me. "He'll listen to me. We won't lose him, okay?"

I nodded, too choked with tears to reply. I walked to the other side of Dad and stroked his head. I looked at him for a few seconds, taking it all in. He looked like he was fading away. It was like he was already dead, but also still dying in front of us.

"Dad? It's Mhairi. If you can hear me, I love you. Please don't leave us, Dad. Don't leave me and Mum. We need you. I'll come home, Dad. Just come back and I'll come home and look after you."

We stood, crying silent tears, holding hands, stroking Dad's face and hands. It was like we were both willing him to react.

A nurse came in.

"Allan needs to be transferred to another hospital. He's still bleeding on the brain, and we don't have the specialist equipment here to stop it. He'll either go to Liverpool or Manchester, depending on where has a bed for him the quickest. The faster he gets to one of these units, the higher chance he will have of making some sort of recovery. He's currently stable but that could change at any time, and if he has another bleed like he had before, he may not make it."

We looked at her, not quite taking it in.

Mum found her voice. "If he hadn't been sent home from A&E the other day, he would have had all the right things done on him and he wouldn't be lying here like this just now though, would he? He should have been scanned. He should have had a lumbar puncture. He should have been kept in. Viral headache? Does this look like a viral headache to you?"

The nurse's eyes were wide open. "Em. No. I know. I can't speak for what happened the other day. I can give you the details if you want to put a complaint in about that."

"Oh, we will be," Mum replied. "Believe you me, we will be. He should not be in this state."

I stepped forward. "If you can get those details, fine. But when will we know about getting him transferred? As you said, it's time-sensitive. He needs to be there now."

"I know. Like I said, we are just waiting for Liverpool or Manchester to phone us as soon as one or another has a bed. Then an ambulance will take Allan."

"Okay, thanks. We will make sure you have our details before we go. You will keep us informed, unlike the other ward, won't you?" I managed a half-smile at her.

She nodded and sloped out the room.

"You okay, Mum?"

"We just need to concentrate on getting your dad back. Did you mean it? Will you come home?"

"Yes, I meant it. I need to go back up the road in the next day or two. Sort things out but then I'll be back down. And I'll go up and down as often as I need to so that I can move back down here. You'll need help, and Dad will too when he's home."

"Thank you. I think we'll have a fight on with the hospital. But they can't get away with this, Mhairi. Look what they've done to him."

"I know, Mum. And they won't. We'll lawyer up, okay? You phone yours and see what we can do. I'll be here with you though, okay? You won't have to do it alone."

I went back up to Fife the next day. A weird thing happens to you when you're faced with trauma. I'd experienced it in boarding school, and with Michael, Nick, and Sarah's dad. A wall goes up. Self-preservation takes over. You know exactly what to do. Fight or flight. In the past, I had done everything possible to get away from a situation and dealt with the after-effects. This time, I knew I had to fight. Fight for Mum and Dad. Everything that had happened before didn't matter at that point. However much I hated the decisions they'd made for me when I was younger, I knew I needed to be with them. Mum was losing her husband and I had become that little Daddy's girl whose dad was never coming back. I needed to move back down to Lancashire. I loved Simon, but at that moment my feelings seemed insignificant, given the newness of the relationship.

"I need to move back home to Lancashire. I know we had plans up here, but I can't leave Mum to deal with everything herself with Dad. I'm sorry, but unless you come with me then I can't be with you. I hope you understand." I felt cruel telling Simon this, but my feelings were overshadowed by the numbness that overcame me. I understood that we would be going our separate ways.

"I'll come with you. Just sort out work. Take enough stuff to keep you going and get back down the road quickly. I'll sort the flat out and follow when I can."

I was astounded, but also grateful. I'd have support, and it meant I could go straight back down to be with Mum and Dad. The next day, I went into work and let my boss know I'd have to resign immediately. He was pretty understanding, considering I'd given them no notice. I was relieved to leave. The Michael/Simon work divide wasn't the nicest atmosphere to be a part of. Soon, I was on a train to Lancashire, in time for Dad to get moved and have his brain surgery. The hospital notified us he'd be moving on September 8 to Manchester, the day after I arrived. They'd been the first to have a bed free. The journey was awful. It was a 50-mile, hour-long drive along busy motorways, filled with lorries criss-crossing through speeding traffic. We followed closely behind the ambulance, as close as Mum dared drive through the chaos. Suddenly, the ambulance's blue lights started to flash. Something was wrong. Mum and I turned to each other in panic.

"Shit! Mum?"

"It's okay. I'll keep up. He'll be okay."

The car accelerated to keep pace with the ambulance. My palms were sweaty, with tears streaming down my cheeks. Mum was on the edge too, but her concentration on staying with Dad kept her in one piece so far as I could see. When we got to the hospital, we found Dad's condition had deteriorated, so they had blue-lighted him the rest of the way. His body was beginning to shut down due to the ongoing bleed. His blood pressure was rocketing again, he was at risk of more fits, and they suspected swelling had started on his brain from all the excess fluid.

Finally, Dad got settled on the neurosurgery unit. He was still unresponsive, his body protecting what life was left in it. The consultant came to speak with us.

"Allan is in bad shape. He's had two catastrophic bleeds, as you know. It's a wonder he's here at all. I can't operate on him until we get him in a more stable condition. It would simply be too dangerous to do it just now. He probably wouldn't survive. The risk of delaying the operation is that he may have an unsurvivable bleed in the meantime. But I think it's the right decision. So realistically, we're looking at Monday for the op."

"Oh lovely. What a nice birthday you'll have, Mum."

"I will if he comes out of it."

We said bye to Dad, and went home. Over the weekend, we made the 100-mile round trip every day, just to check on how he was doing. Luckily, Dad remained stable over the weekend and the consultants looking after him made the decision to operate on him on the Monday. When Monday came around, our silence said everything we needed it to. Mum and I barely spoke a word to each other from when we got out of bed. We just needed to get to the hospital and wait for news. We spent hours in the small waiting room, until eventually the consultant came to see us.

"Allan came through the operation fine. He is one tough man; I can tell you. I put a new kind of coil in to stop the bleed. It's platinum and should do the job nicely. It will stay there indefinitely. He's got a drain from his brain to take off the excess fluid build-up from surgery, and another one from his stomach. These can be removed in a couple of days. I've also had to put a temporary external shunt in from his brain, down to his stomach because his brain isn't getting rid of the fluid like it should. He will need a permanent shunt fitted soon. He's not out of the woods yet, but he is in a better state than he was. He could still have another bleed. It's just a waiting game. You can go in to see him now. Just one at a time though. Follow me, Joyce."

Mum followed the consultant, while I sat and waited. Then it was my turn. I walked through to the double doors into Dad's room and pushed the bell. The buzzer sounded, and I pushed open the doors. If I thought Dad looked ill before with all the wires hanging out of him, it was worse now. His head was bandaged, with tubes coming out from under them, some leading back under the covers, and some leading to a bag which was slowly filling with blood and cerebral fluid. He had another bag coming out from under the sheets, filling up with gastric fluid and more blood. I fought back the tears as I held his hand.

"Dad? It's Mhairi."

His eyes flickered open, revealing a glazed expression, aware that there was someone, something there.

"Hi. You're back. I'm here, Dad. It's Mhairi."

I repeated myself, hoping for a glimmer of recognition from him. But there was none. I tried to stay strong and to keep the tears hidden, but I couldn't do it. It was too much. He looked so helpless. I leant over and kissed his cheek and felt a light squeeze on my hand. That gave me hope that he at least knew who I was, even if he couldn't tell me in his own words.

That night, Mum went to visit our neighbour, Caroline, whom we'd known in Saudi Arabia. She was gone for hours, while I cuddled up on the couch with Glen, our beefy yellow Labrador, and Kirsty, our hyperactive six-month-old yellow retriever. They were my security blanket. I hadn't shut the curtains, preferring instead to look out over the field in front of the house. Glen started growling his deep, throaty sound, then Kirsty started yapping. I looked out the window to see mum slithering down the window. I ran outside to get her, thinking that she was ill.

"Mum! Are you okay?" I screamed, as I caught her wobbling back and forth.

"I. Am. Abslutly. Fin." She looked round at me with a toothy grin, and laughed through clenched teeth, spraying saliva. The stench of wine knocked me backwards.

"Aw, Jeez-o, Mother! Had a little drink, have you? Come on, in we go." I helped her in and sat her down at the kitchen table, then put the kettle on.

"I only had one. Fell off the chair."

Mum is not a drinker. Half a glass of wine and she'll be pole-dancing round the closest bird table. With all the stress of the past couple of weeks, the glass of red that she claimed to have had had gotten her paralytic. She cradled her cup of tea whilst she sobered up a bit.

A little later, she said, "Right!" then got up, put on the rubber gloves that were draped over the tap, opened the fridge, and started pulling everything out.

"Mum, what are you doing? It's past midnight. You cannae be doing that just now."

"I can. I have to, Mhairi! I can't go to bed just now. And the fridge needs it."

She wasn't wrong, so I got a spare pair of gloves, and we emptied the fridge and started cleaning. We didn't get to bed until well after two in the morning.

CHAPTER 17

Dad continued to improve over the next week or so until he was moved down to a general medical ward from the high dependency ward. Mum and I went to the hospital every day, making the 100-mile round trip without a second thought. Hope Hospital was like a second home for us in that we spent as much time there as we did at home. The ward Dad was in had three other patients, all in a similar condition. He kept improving, and the more time passed, the less likely it became that he was going to have another bleed on the brain. He was now opening his eyes and making little movements with his lips, but he still had a glazed expression, and no sounds apart from the odd squeak came from his mouth. Mum and I would sit for hours, talking to him, watching him sleep, showing him familiar things, all in a vain attempt to get him to say or see something familiar. It was heartbreaking to live through. One day, we went in and noticed he looked a little droopy. I went straight to his notes at the bottom of the bed.

"His BP's okay, Mum. Temp's up a bit. And his GCS has dipped back down again. Something's not right." I flicked through the pages. "What's this?" I read the sheet in disbelief. "Mum? He's got MRSA. How the hell has he got that? He's not even being barrier-nursed, and there's no signs up anywhere. And he's still on a ward with these guys."

Dad had caught the hospital superbug, Methicillin-resistant Staphylococcus aureus (MRSA), and as Mum and I knew from working with Dad in the nursing home, there should have been signs up to let people know he had it, gloves and aprons should have been provided and if available, he should have been moved to a room of his own to prevent spreading the bug to anybody else.

"You are joking! Mhairi, his drainage bags are practically empty. He's got a blockage in that shunt. He must have." I looked over to the drainage bag coming from the bandage around Dad's head wound. The bags should have had some fluid in them to show the drains were working properly and preventing liquid from building up in his head which could have caused more brain damage. Instead, his drainage bag was empty, which meant there was a blockage preventing liquid from coming out.

Mum was fuming. We should have been told when we arrived in the ward about his MRSA. At the very least, there should have been a warning. His empty drainage bags not having any liquid in them should have been picked up as an emergency.

"That's it. Wait here!" Mum flew out of the ward. I saw her shaking her head at the nurse and pointing to the office, which they promptly disappeared into. Five minutes later, she returned. "Come on, we're leaving, or I'll smack someone."

After a few minutes of silence in the car, Mum let me know that she'd pulled the nurse into the office and given her a lecture on infection control. She'd also suggested there was a problem with Dad's shunt that should have been picked up on. We were well versed in it, Mum and I having worked in medical settings for so many years between us, and we'd had the best teacher there was – Dad. When we got home, there were three messages on the answering machine from the nurse asking Mum to call the ward. She didn't return the calls. In the morning, she phoned to check how Dad was doing, and it was a different nurse that answered.

"Well," Mum said after she'd hung up. "Your dad's now being barrier-nursed. He was pulled into surgery last night to get internal shunts put in because we were right. The ones that he had were blocked. How many times are they going to mess him up? We need to look after him, Mhairi. We can't leave him anywhere to rot."

"I promise, Mum. We'll do it between us. We'll see he's looked after properly."

***

In October 2005, the doctors decided Dad didn't need to be on the ward any more. There was nothing else they could do for him. He'd improved to the extent that he was able to eat and drink, with a lot of help, and he was able to be transferred into a wheelchair. He moved closer to home, to a little cottage hospital just outside of Blackpool. It was mainly used for rehabilitating elderly patients before they went home or into a nursing home. The ward Dad was put in had three bays of six people, all in a similar condition. Every day for the next few weeks, sometimes twice a day, Mum and I would go to see Dad, help with his care, and just sit with him and talk to him. He now had more animation in his eyes, and he'd reach out and touch us and move his lips, but still no words came out. Just the odd 'Ugh' and 'Ooh'. He seemed to have reached a plateau in his recovery, and there was talk of him being moved to a nursing home, because nobody on the ward thought he could be looked after at home. It was like they were just giving up on him getting any better and just settling for how he was at that moment being as good as he was ever going to get.

Mum had been signed off sick from work since Dad took ill in early September. Luckily, she was getting full sick pay. Dad was only getting statutory sick pay as there wasn't a healthcare scheme at his job. I hadn't even looked for a job yet, and it was now December. Simon had finally tied up all the loose ends, packed the flat up in Fife and moved down. We both managed to get part-time jobs in a small call centre near Preston, selling mobile phone contract extensions. It was monotonous, and we worked on a commission basis, but it was something to help with the mounting bills and overdue mortgage payments at Mum and Dad's house. Even though we were all clubbing together, things were tighter than ever. Mum and I knew we might need to make adaptations to the house if we were ever going to get Dad home, which meant more costs, but we were determined to bring him home to look after him. Having worked for years in hospitals and nursing homes we knew that, with all the goodwill in the world, staff shortages and cutbacks affected patient care. We didn't want that for Dad. It became apparent that the rehabilitation care he was getting at the hospital was basic and lacked the speciality resources that he needed for his brain haemorrhage. In preparation for beginning to look at nursing homes, we'd been assigned a social worker, Beth.

"There is one other option," she said. "There's a specialised inpatient rehabilitation centre in Bury, near Manchester. They deal with brain injury rehabilitation for adults. The only drawback is that it is privately funded. Now Allan may be a candidate to get that paid for him by the local primary care trust and I can certainly put him forward, but if they don't agree then it is a question of private funding which would be £20,000."

Mum and I just looked at each other. We couldn't get that sort of money together. We'd have to sell the house.

"Do it," I said.

"Put the request in," Mum said. "He is not going into a home."

A few days later, Beth returned. "I'm sorry, but they won't authorise the funds to send Allan to rehab. They recognised that he was an ideal candidate, but they just can't do it at the moment."

"What do you mean they won't do it?" I asked.

"You said it yourself, Beth, he's an ideal candidate. Why won't they send him?" Mum asked.

"It comes down to budgets and whether they have the funds. We could try again in the new financial year, but they just won't do it right now."

"Like hell they won't," I said. "Watch me phone the head of the primary care trust. What's the number?"

"I can't give that out," Beth said.

"Fine, I will find it myself. My dad is going to that rehab unit. Nobody else is going to fuck up his health," I replied to her very quietly but made sure every word was as clear as a bell.

"You do know we're in touch with medical negligence lawyers in Manchester? Allan should not be in the state he's in. It wouldn't be a good idea to refuse him the care he deserves after it was a hospital error that got him there in the first place. I think we'll give the news a wee phone when we get home too, won't we, Mhairi?" Mum said her piece and I nodded in agreement before we walked away, leaving Beth standing there.

That night we went home, and Mum contacted the local news. They sent a journalist the next morning. That night, we were on the six o'clock and the ten o' clock news. We felt sure the report would make a difference, but two days later we still hadn't heard anything. On the third day, I was at work but I couldn't concentrate on anything other than my dad, destined to be stuck the way he was. On my lunch break, I managed to find the name and number of the CEO of the local primary care trust, and by some miracle I got put through to him.

"Good afternoon. It's Mhairi Hutt here. Do you know that surname at all?" I asked.

"Afternoon. No. Should I?" he quipped.

"My dad is Allan Hutt. Gilbert Allan Hutt, actually. You refused to fund him for a private rehab place in Bury. He had a brain haemorrhage. The hospital was at fault."

"Ah yes. I do remember. We can't just fund everyone that asks for the money."

"Did you see the local news the other night?" I asked.

He laughed. "No. I was in London with my family. Look, I'm sorry I can't fund your dad, but we need to make sure everyone is cost-effective."

My mouth fell open, and I saw red. Wrong answer!

"What did you just say to me? Cost-effective? I'm glad you were able to go away with your family to London. I can't do that because my dad is currently lying in a hospital bed because of medical negligence which, by the way, we now have a team of lawyers behind us looking into. I'll tell you something. I have been a patient, a carer and a relative. Have you?"

"No, but I ..."

"No, thought not. Would you refuse any of your family twenty grand to give them the best chance of recovering from a medical mistake? I don't think so. If anybody deserves that money to go to rehab it's my dad. He's been a nurse for nearly forty years. I hope one of these days your family's lives are in someone else's hands to play God with. See what decision you'd make then. Are their lives worth twenty grand? You make me sick!"

I hung up the phone. I was crying, shaking. I felt nauseous. I chain-smoked three cigarettes, before going back to work twenty minutes late. I didn't even hear the dressing down I got from the manager. I didn't care. The next morning, we got the news that Dad had been granted the funding to go to rehab. The CEO had apparently had a change of heart.

CHAPTER 18

Dad was moved to the private rehab unit within days. He had his own room, which was simple but functional. It looked just like any other hospital room, with its magnolia walls, hospital bed, and over-bed table on wheels. He had the standard bedside locker with a cubby hole and a cupboard and a single pine-veneered wardrobe next to the sink. His treatment began right away. He had a speech therapist, a physiotherapist, an occupational therapist, carers, doctors, nurses, and Beth.

There was no plan for how long he would be there. The only plan was to get some improvement out of him so that he could have some quality of life – to get him talking again, moving a bit more, and make sure he was on all the right medication for the future.

Dad had only been in the unit a couple of weeks when we started to notice small improvements. With each new visit, he seemed a little brighter and more relaxed, as though he realised that he was coming out of the fog. But by Christmas, he still hadn't spoken. We took him home for Christmas Day, but it was like having a ghost at the table. Dad and I were usually the ones who put the tree up together. It felt pointless celebrating Christmas like this. He was alive, but there was an emptiness, like a discarded hermit crab shell. He kept staring at Simon, and then at the ring on my finger that had been put on it just days before. There had been no big proposal, nor any traditional asking of my dad for his approval. Simon and I were standing in the kitchen alone when he suddenly got down on one knee. He pulled a ring box from his jeans pocket and then just a simply said, "Will you marry me, please?" He opened the box to reveal a gold ring with a little diamond shining at me.

"Yeah, I will", I said.

Engagement, marriage, a future – it all seemed so trivial with Dad lying in a bed, unaware of anything going on. I loved Simon and he was there for me, had been since the beginning of Dad's illness. It was a safe decision with little fuss, and I couldn't see a future without Simon in it.

***

One day in January 2006, Mum and I went in to see Dad. He was usually asleep in the afternoons. But he must have heard us, as his eyes pinged open when we approached the bed.

"Hello," he said, as clear as a bell. "What are you two doing here?"

Mum and I just looked at each other in disbelief.

"Hi Dad. It's Mum and Mhairi," I practically squeaked.

"I know who you are. But what are you doing here in Bordeaux? And where are the four dogs and three cats? I can't find them."

"Bordeaux?" Mum said. "Allan, you're in Bury in the rehab unit. We only have two dogs and they're back home."

"Don't be silly, Joyce. This is Bordeaux, and the dogs and cats must be running about somewhere. Why are you here?"

Mum and I sat with him for ages, explaining to him what had happened over the past four months. When the nurse arrived, she was amazed that he'd suddenly started speaking. It was like the mains had been switched back on, and everything was powering up. Apparently, he'd been saying the odd half-word or two in his speech therapy sessions, but nothing substantial like he was coming out with now. Admittedly, it was completely senseless, but he was talking again, and that could only be a step in the right direction. From that day on, there were gradual improvements to Dad's speech and mobility every time I saw him. He would come out with more words, and the little things he would say would make more sense, like asking how I was, or what I'd been doing. He was slow, and the words didn't come easily, but they did come eventually. It was such a relief to see some of his character coming back.

While things with Dad were improving through the rest of January, February and into March, things with the house were in dire straits. Mum's sick pay was coming to an end, meaning she would need to go back to work full-time. The bank had paused the mortgage payments on the house for us, but they were going to restart them, and Mum's salary would barely cover the new repayments. We needed to sell the house. We didn't want to stay in the area, in case anything happened to Dad's head again, and he was sent to the hospital that had misdiagnosed him. Mum and Dad had always planned to move home to Scotland when they retired, but further north than Fife. Mum and I decided Inverness was the place. If we bought a house on the outskirts, we'd be close to one of the local doctor's surgeries and away from the hospital that had failed Dad, but it would fulfil Mum and Dad's retirement plans for retiring up north.

We told the rehabilitation unit what we were planning, but they gave us no information about transferring Dad's care when we moved. When we tried to discuss it, we were given only vague acknowledgements of our plans, and nothing more. It was strange.

By April, we'd sold the house. After a couple of trips to Inverness, Mum and I had picked our new home. It was a four-bedroom dormer bungalow straight out of the eighties, in a cul-de-sac on the edge of Inverness. It had a built-in stone fireplace that ran the length of the wall, the kind which you could put your TV in one corner and the customary chintzy vase full of pink silk roses in the other corner. All the interior wood was dark, and the doors had round brass handles on them. The staircase had open treads and big horizontal slats of wood running up the side. The house would need a lot of work to make it accessible for Dad, but we had the room to do it. We would be moving up in June. When we notified the rehab unit of our moving date, their response was no longer vague.

"There's really nothing more we can do for Allan anyway. We think he'd be best placed in a nursing home. You won't be able to look after him at home," one of the doctors said. There was that sentence again – 'You won't be able to look after him at home'.

"You've all done a great job with my dad. He's improved so much but there is no way on this planet that he will be going into a nursing home. He either stays here or he comes home before we can get him up to Inverness. Nowhere else."

"We really can't keep him here. We've done all we can. Maybe we should have a team meeting to discuss the best path forward."

"What a good idea. But I'm telling you now, it's either here or home. There is no path that leads to a nursing home. I will fight you all the way on that."

A couple of weeks later, Mum, Dad and I sat outside a room waiting for the meeting to start. We were called through and I wheeled Dad into the large room which had triple bay windows at the other end. The room was set up as a conference room with a rectangle made up of desks, and about fifteen chairs. Most were filled with the entire multidisciplinary team who had looked after Dad for the past few months. There were the nurses, doctors, all the therapists, the centre manager, and Beth. We were heavily outnumbered, and from the outset we were up against it.

One by one, the team who had been involved in Dad's care gave us progress reports from their specific area of expertise. There was no denying, it was impressive. He'd gone from a near-vegetative state to being able to feed himself and comprehend and respond to simple questions. He was mobile enough to help get himself washed and dressed by moving his arms and legs when asked to but that was the extent of his abilities, and he was still doubly incontinent and needed 24-hour care and supervision. He wouldn't be able to be left alone and didn't have the mental capacity to make decisions for himself. To all intents and purposes, he was a child. The unit manager spoke to us first.

"Allan really can't be discharged to home," she said. "The best place for him would be some sort of residential unit where his needs would be met round the clock."

"I don't think so," Mum said. "We are more than capable of looking after him at home. In fact, we'd be with him all the time, so he'd have more supervision."

"Yes," answered Beth, the social worker, "but you'll need supplies like pads, and equipment like a commode and wheelchair and in the future maybe a hoist. Your home might need adapting to suit Allan's needs. Have you thought of that?"

"Yes, we've thought of that," Mum replied. "Anything Allan needs, we will get for him. And there are care packages that you can source for us, aren't there? If he needs to be discharged from here before then?"

"Mrs Hutt," Beth answered. "It's all very well you wanting Allan at home. We understand you've all had a rough time. But I can't just magic a care package out of thin air. The finances simply won't allow it. A home would be better."

"Listen to me, Beth," Mum replied as her face reddened and her voice shook. "I don't care if you need to walk the streets of Blackpool to get the finances together to get Allan home. If you are kicking him out of here, he is not, nor ever will be, going into any kind of home."

Mum got up and walked out of the meeting. I looked at Dad and squeezed his hand a little tighter. He smirked and rolled his eyes. The room was deathly silent for a few seconds.

The unit manager spoke. "Mhairi, we understand your mum is upset."

"I'll stop you there," I interrupted. "I recognise the amazing job you have all done, and I'll be forever grateful to you all, and yes, it seems Dad has reached a plateau here. Do you really think stuffing him in a nursing home because the funding might not be available would be the best thing for him? I've had this funding argument before, remember. That's why he's here in the first place. If it's the same guy who's responsible for authorizing the funding, Beth, I have absolutely no problem in giving him another call. However, I do not think that moving my dad anywhere for eight weeks would benefit anybody, most of all my dad. It would take as long to get everything in place and only confuse him. If you are open to it, I would like to ask my dad what he wants. It is, after all, his life we are discussing."

There were nods all-round the table.

"Dad?"

He looked at me, and I felt his fingers tighten round mine.

"Do you want to go to a nursing home?"

He looked at me for a couple of seconds and I thought he might not have understood me properly, and my idea would have failed. Then, he shook his head. He let go of my hand, looked round the room, and started shaking his finger from side to side.

"Okay. I think that's a no. Dad, would you like to come home to Inverness?"

He looked me in the eyes, his own eyes welling up. He put his arms around me, nodding his head. I put my arms round him, fighting back my own tears.

"Okay, Dad. No problem. You're coming home." I looked back to our audience. "I think that says it all, don't you? I'm going to take Dad out to Mum while you discuss his care for the next eight weeks. Thank you."

I got up and wheeled Dad out to see Mum, who was still wiping the tears from her cheeks.

"He's coming home, Mum. He wants to be at home," I said to her.

The three of us held onto each other, shedding happy tears.

CHAPTER 19

We completed our move to Inverness on June 6, 2006. Two weeks later, Mum and Simon went down to Bury to collect Dad and finally bring him home. The house was big enough, but it wasn't great for Dad. The doorways weren't quite wide enough for Dad's wheelchair, so it meant there had to be two of us to walk him through doors when he was too tired to try to walk himself. There were stairs to the front and back of the house that needed to have ramps fitted and the bathroom he was going to be able to access had a shower with a high step up to it. Although Dad was managing to stay continent most of the time, and even wash himself with supervision we knew the house could be so much better for him if we got it remodelled to accommodate all our needs.

Although the clinical negligence case was ongoing, and it looked likely that we would win the case, we were far away from a settlement, so Mum and Dad couldn't afford the renovations. Simon had found a job in a supermarket, and I'd started working in a bookmaker's, and we were both on reasonable money. We offered to buy into the house to give Mum and Dad the money to pay for the work. It would mean taking on a mortgage, but it was only a temporary measure. We'd own the house while the work was going on, until we could pay off the mortgage. It suited us all, so the renovations commenced.

The upstairs, which Simon and I would occupy, was transformed from two double bedrooms with a little shower room to a living room, double bedroom, and ensuite bathroom on one side of the house and on the other was a double bedroom, single bedroom, and a shower room.

Downstairs went from having a single and a double bedroom to having a double with ensuite bathroom, a study, another double bedroom, and a wet room, all with wide doors for Dad getting round. The old, dark kitchen was ripped out to make way for light grey units. The old fireplace got ripped out in the living room and we had decking built with French doors to make getting out to the garden easy for Dad.

By September, Simon and I had started planning our wedding for the following August. We would have it in Kirkcaldy, where most of our family lived, and it would be a triple celebration incorporating our wedding, Mum and Dad's silver wedding anniversary and Dad's sixtieth birthday. We had a lot to celebrate. In my mind, Simon was the one for me. The only incident we'd ever fallen out over was when I had asked him to help clear rooms before the work got done. He had been playing on his PlayStation, and I must have asked him about four or five times to come and help me move boxes. My moods were all over the place, for some reason.

"Simon, would you please just turn that bloody game off and come and help me!" I shouted.

I wished I hadn't. The next thing I knew, a games controller went whistling past my head, and crashed into the door. I had sudden flashes of Michael and the breadknife, and Nick throwing me against the wall, as Simon got up and stormed past me. Was it my fault because I'd shouted at him? Should I have just left him to play his game, and done the jobs myself? But then I thought, Should I have just cleaned that grill for Michael? Maybe he wouldn't have thrown the knife at me. Should I have just given Nick that money? Then he wouldn't have thrown me against the wall. I just stood there and cried.

Was Simon even right for me? When I met him, I was in a bad place. I'd lost my identity – I didn't really know who I was at all. The last time I had felt 'normal' was when I was ten. Nearly losing Dad had forced me to be strong for him and Mum. When Simon had come along, it was like finding a weighted blanket at first. The safety and security of him was refreshing, but now I was doubting myself.

Three weeks later, I had debilitating stomach cramps and started getting a metal taste in my mouth. For a day or two, I had little spots of blood, then the familiar heavy blood loss and huge clots, as I suffered miscarriage number five. I was shaking with pain and had clammy skin from the stress my body was under. I went to the doctor, and I was referred to gynaecology to start infertility investigations. I was given tranexamic acid for my heavy bleeding and told to keep taking it for my usual monthly periods to stop the heavy blood loss.

"Just rest up for a day or two. The pills should help. Take paracetamol and just keep trying. You'll hear from gynaecology with an appointment," the doctor told me. It was as simple as that for him. Take a pill, get back on the horse. I'd lost five babies, and it was getting too much.

I threw myself into my work. I took any training they would give me over the next few months. I travelled from Inverness to Aberdeen, Glasgow, and Edinburgh to work my way up to management level. I began training new employees and worked any extra shifts I could. When I wasn't at work, I was helping with Dad at home and walking the two dogs. I barely slept, and my weight plummeted from ten-and-a-half stone to eight stone seven.

In March 2007, we got the news that my nana had terminal lung cancer. She only had six weeks to live. Mum and Dad went down to Kirkcaldy so that Mum could nurse her at home, I went down on my days off to give Mum a helping hand.

"Come and help me, Mhairi," Nana said. She was such an independent person, that I was slightly taken aback.

Nana never asked for help and was always meticulous with her appearance. She would wear a mid-calf length navy blue skirt with nude tights and navy-blue court shoes with a modest two-inch heel. She'd wear a little blouse or fine-knit jumper with elbow-length sleeves in pastel shades, cream or white. When she was cleaning, she would always have a pinny tied round her waist, covered in cigarette burns, even though she always denied that she smoked. Her grey hair was always fine and bouncy from having her curlers in, those little pink or blue ones with bristles round them.

Now, in her long white, sleeveless nightdress, I could see her bones protruding through her paper-thin skin. Her hair was matted to her head from her days lying in bed. She held onto me as I helped her onto the commode at the side of her bed. I got a basin of warm water and her bar of imperial leather soap and washed her, then put a fresh nightie on her and gave her hair a brush. I sprayed her signature lavender spray on her wrists, as she sat in silence, holding on to me. When I finished, she gave a gummy smile, and put her arms round me like a child.

She looked up. "Thank you, hen. I'd only let you or your mum do that. I feel a bit fresher now. Listen, I don't think I'll make your wedding in August, but your papa knows what to do, so he'll give you a wee cheque from us, okay?"

Nana and Papa had been married for over sixty years and it was always Nana who organised cards and presents for birthdays and other special occasions. It came as no surprise that she'd thought about an occasion that was over four months away.

"Nana, you don't need to worry about that just now."

"It's done. Now, in the cupboard above the cooker in the teapot at the back, there's a packet of cigarettes. You take them because I don't think I'll have them now." I couldn't help but let out a laugh. "Also, I know you're going to Crete soon. Could you look for my cousin Jim? James. He went to

Greece in the war, possibly Crete and never came back. I don't know where he is."

"Of course I will, Nana. I'll look him up before I go."

That was the last time I saw my nana. I went home to Inverness to go back to work. A few days later, Mum phoned.

"Now your papa's in the hospital. Daft old bugger thought he'd tidy the garden and he fell and broke his hip. He's in the hospital but he'll be fine. Great timing!"

"Just what you don't need, Mum. At least he'll be okay, and he'll be out soon. Put Nana on the phone will you." I waited while Mum took the phone to Nana's room.
"Nana? Can you hear me?" I heard a murmur. "I found Jim, Nana. I looked on the computer and found war grave records. Jim was listed as a member of the Black Watch. He was in the Battle of Crete when he died on May 20, 1941. I won't be able to see his memorial this time because it's in Athens. But I'll have a wee drink on the beach for him, okay? Love you, Nana."

I heard another murmur.

It was night-time on April 21 when Mum phoned me to tell me that Nana had died. Her funeral was held a few days before I went to Crete. I had a good few drinks in Crete for both Nana and Jim.

I didn't cope well after Nana's death. I was trying to organise a wedding, but also mourning Nana, and I hadn't stopped thinking about losing yet another baby. I went back to the doctor with depression, but they were reluctant to do anything because I was on the waiting list for gynaecology, and they thought it might be hormonal. Instead, they took blood samples to check for my immunity to rubella, my iron levels, and my progesterone levels. Unsurprisingly, the test results indicated that I was borderline anaemic, and I wasn't ovulating properly. I was told to wait for my hospital appointment, start taking folic acid, and advised that I would probably feel better in a couple of months' time after all the stress of planning my wedding was over.

On August 7, I married Simon in a hotel in Kirkcaldy, as well as celebrating Mum and Dad's silver wedding anniversary and Dad's sixtieth birthday, in front of over a hundred family members and friends. My papa had made a good recovery from his broken hip and although he wasn't able to walk more than a few steps unaided, he was there in his wheelchair. My dad on the other hand had improved with his mobility so much that he walked me down the aisle, something that a year earlier I had thought could never happen. I stood in front of Simon in my long white dress, with its sweetheart neckline, lace bodice and silk skirt that was plumped out with a multi-layered petticoat. My delicate veil, laced with pearls, was fixed in place with a diamanté tiara, and covered my face.

It was surreal. Half the people there were there for Mum and Dad, and had never really featured in my life. I felt like it wasn't really my day, but another part of me was relishing it. As Dad gave me away, and I recited my vows, I cried tears of happiness. I was finally in a safe place in my life. I had Mum and Dad, who needed me, and I had Simon, who wanted me, and whom I trusted and felt safe with.

The next day, we sat and opened our cards and gifts, I saw my papa's writing on an envelope. It was a cheque for £100. My name and the amount were written in Nana's handwriting on the cheque, and Papa had signed the card from them both. It was like she'd been there on the day.

After the wedding, Papa's health started to fail. He could walk short distances with a Zimmer frame, but he was getting noticeably slower, and struggling to hold on to the sides of the frame. He had bad emphysema and struggled to breath properly. In late November, he started getting shaky, to the point where things would fly out of his hands when he was trying to use them, like his inhaler or his old CB radio. We would laugh about it, and I'd pretend we were playing baseball, but it was only to keep the sadness away.

On the last visit from the doctor, Papa was told that his kidneys were failing, and he didn't have long left. A couple of days later, he went to bed for the last time. He fell asleep, and three days later, on December 9, he died, with us at his bedside. Even the dogs were watching over him. I couldn't bring myself to go to the funeral, which I regret. I'd had enough death and sadness, and I couldn't face it, having to make small talk. In a little over a year, I'd lost my fifth baby, and both my grandparents. It was too much to take.

In December, I finally got to see a gynaecologist.

"I'm diagnosing you with extremely severe dysmenorrhoea – basically your periods are unbearably painful. But I think you might have endometriosis. The only way that can be confirmed is by having a laparoscopy. If you're okay with that, I'll put you on the waiting list. It's only three to six months, so not too long. I'll take some bloods from you today and send them away to check all your hormones and iron. In the meantime, just keep trying for a baby, keep taking painkillers, and manage as best you can. There's nothing else we can do at this point."

With that, he proceeded to drain my arm of eight vials of blood, then sent me on my way. It was the first time endometriosis had ever been mentioned to me.

When I got home, I looked it up. The appointment had been so matter-of-fact and quick that I hadn't asked any questions. The more I read, the more sense it made: painful periods, vomiting and diarrhoea during menstruation, multiple miscarriages, heavy bleeding, depression, mood swings, abdominal pain, shoulder pain – you name it, at some point during my menstrual life I'd had it. As far as I was concerned, I'd found my answer, but there was no cure. It was a disease to be 'managed'.

I decided to try and put everything to the back of my mind and try to enjoy Christmas and the New Year. I was newly married, had a good job, and Dad was still improving. Our medical negligence lawyers had started putting our case forward through the courts and, though nothing would move quickly, it was looking very promising. By the end of January 2008, I realised my period was late. This time, I realised I was pregnant. A test revealed a very faint, positive result.

I went to the fridge and took some ham out of a half-eaten packet. It tasted like metal, and I realised that must be my pregnancy trait. Apparently, my mum's had been a sudden dislike for mince and tatties – Nana had made them for her one day, and she felt sick at the sight of them. Nana realised she must have been pregnant again. Mine was metal ham. I spoke to the doctor.

"I understand you think you're pregnant. We'll let the hospital know, and you'll get a scan at twelve weeks to check your progress. Continue to take your folic acid," she said.

"Can I not get an early scan? I've had five miscarriages already. I'm a bit worried."

"I'm sorry. We don't routinely offer early scans unless there's a good reason. I'm sure you'll be fine."

But I wasn't. A week later, I had awful cramping, and the all-too-familiar blood and clotting that meant my body was rejecting baby number six. I called the doctor, and was told to go in immediately. I lay on the table, my stomach in shreds, crying as I was prodded and poked by a man with a strange face and a crappy bedside manner.

"You're guarding your stomach," he said. "I can't get a proper feel. Can you relax a little?"

"No wonder I'm guarding my stomach! I'm having a miscarriage and you're not exactly gentle." I didn't care that I was abrupt, and I just turned my face away whilst he had another prod.

"I'll give you painkillers. Just rest up for a day again. You should be fine after that." I took my prescription, got my tablets, and went home. I was getting fed up with being told I'd be fine. Keep trying. Here's some codeine, that'll fix it. I was fast realising that I couldn't keep going like this.

CHAPTER 20

About a week before I was due to go into hospital for the investigative surgery, Simon and I were sitting together.

"I'm going to join the police force. I've already sent the initial application off and if I'm successful I'll start later in the year," he said.

"Well, I didn't see that coming. How long have you been thinking about that? It's not something you've ever mentioned."

"Yeah, I just fancy it. It'll mean I'll be away Monday to Friday for a few months, but it will be worth it."

I was happy for him. It was the first time he'd showed any real gusto for something that was his and his alone. I did wonder how he would manage, though, as he was a quiet man, bordering on shy at times. I remember thinking that maybe it would help him become less shy. I was nervous for him, but I put it to the back of my mind as I prepared to go into hospital.

***

I woke up on the gynaecological ward in Inverness hospital, seeing blurry figures of nurses in the ward, in late March 2008. The buzz of the hospital ward confused me as I came to my senses after the general anaesthetic. I saw nurses walking about, and then saw Simon sitting next to me and realised I was awake after my operation. I had an oxygen mask on and was hooked up to the blood pressure and pulse monitor, and I had a drip.

A little later, the consultant appeared at my bedside.

"Your laparoscopy went well," he said. "I found your right fallopian tube was stuck to your right ovary, and you had a two-inch chocolate cyst there too. I drained that. Your left ovary is stuck to your pelvic side wall. I found signs of endometriosis all over your uterus and ovaries, on your bladder, bowel, and pouch of Douglas. I've drained the cyst and scraped some of the endometriosis away and flushed out your tubes. That should ease your symptoms for now. I'd like to keep you in overnight just to get those IV antibiotics into you and monitor your recovery overnight. If all goes well, you can go home tomorrow, and I'll see you in clinic in a couple of weeks."

I was still too out of it to take anything in properly at that moment. Over the next couple of weeks, I had the time I needed to digest everything he'd said. At least I had an answer for my unnaturally painful periods and multiple miscarriages.

For two weeks I dosed myself up on co-codamol and ibuprofen four times a day. When I attended my post-operative follow-up appointment, I asked the doctor if there were any options to help me manage better.

"I can give you more painkillers," he said. "But there is no cure for endometriosis. It is a condition that you will have for life. You can try the Mirena coil or the pill, or you can have a baby."

"Are those seriously my options? We have been trying to have a baby, but I can't seem to carry past a couple of months."

"Yes, that will be the endometriosis."

"I really don't want to go on contraception. Every pill I've tried has given me some sort of side effect. I've had migraines, some of them make my periods heavier and even more painful. And I don't want a coil all stuck up inside of me."

"Well, we can try a drug called clomiphene then. It helps stimulate your ovaries into producing more eggs and given your right ovary isn't working fully because of the endometriosis and the cyst, I'd say it's worth a try. There is a risk of hyperstimulation of the ovaries which can lead to hospitalisation, but it's very low. I'll give you the prescription, but you'll need blood tests first to check your progesterone and oestrogen levels, or to detect a pregnancy. You can start the clomiphene any time after you've had your bloods taken once a month for two months in a row."

"Okay. My husband is going away to police college shortly though, so I'll start taking them when he's back."

***

Simon went away to police college at the beginning of August. He was away from Sunday afternoons until Friday nights. Following the operation, my periods had calmed down a little. I was still in severe pain, and they were still heavy, but they were more bearable. At the end of August, I was late. I couldn't believe it. It was the first time I had consciously realised I was late and that I could be pregnant. I bought pregnancy tests on my lunch break from work one day. I went to a different chemist from my usual one, and bought five. I thought, Maybe it's a faulty batch of tests so I'll check another chemist. That night when I got home from work, I took one. It came back positive. Then I took another, and another, until I'd used up four. I looked at them, all lined up on the bathroom worktop, all showing I was pregnant. I phoned Simon.

"I'm pregnant! I took four tests, and they're all positive. The operation must have worked, Simon. I'm actually pregnant!"

"Oh my god, that's amazing. I'm so happy for you. Listen I need to go now but I'll speak to you later. I'm getting ready for our night out. Speak later."

I could hear the muffled voices in the background and was a little hurt that he hadn't shown more interest, but he had his own stuff going on, so I tried my best to deal with things on my own. I had Mum, and to some degree I had Dad too. He knew enough of what was going on to ask how I was and if I was feeling okay, but I needed Simon, and he was physically and emotionally, absent.

I went about my days rubbing my tummy, talking to the little seed growing inside of me. Looking on the internet at nursery furniture and prams and looking up all the advice for being a good mummy. I'd always liked the name April for a girl, or Ben for a boy. I thought about my suitcase of baby clothes packed away in the loft that I could finally get out and use on my own child. My belly was swelling a little, and I was sick most nights. I was finally allowing myself to hope. I didn't even mind being sick because, for me, it was the best thing to ever happen to me.

I only experienced the happiness of knowing I was pregnant for two weeks. I started getting twinges in my stomach, and that acrid metal taste came on my tongue, even without the ham. I phoned the doctors, and they said just rest and take painkillers. It was probably my womb stretching. I took their advice and went to bed with excruciating cramps. I woke up the next morning to a bloody bed. I went to the bathroom, sat on the toilet, and felt a mass come out of me. I knew what it was. I burst into tears and gave out a long, painful moan. I was alone in the house, and I couldn't even phone Simon, because he was in lectures. I phoned the doctor again, still crying.

"I'm sorry, Mhairi," the female doctor said. "It does sound as though you've had another miscarriage. I don't think there's any point bringing you in or booking you in to the hospital. You seem to know what you're talking about, and you've still got your painkillers. My best advice is to rest. If you need a sick note for work for a while, I will write one, no problem. If you start getting sharp pains or heavy bleeding, then phone back and we'll get you in."

The doctor was sympathetic as she gave me her advice. When I hung up the phone, I lay back on the couch and clutched my stomach. Mum and Dad looked after me when they got back home from their outing: lots of cups of tea, plenty of cuddles and making sure I was resting. I just cuddled the dogs on the couch. There's something about a good snuggle from a dog that makes everything bearable, if only for a while. I finally got hold of Simon later that night.

"I lost the baby. I'm so sorry. I don't know what happened."

"I … I don't know what to say. I told everyone I was gonna be a dad. I'll need to untell them now, won't I."

"I'm sorry, Simon. I don't know what else to say. There's nothing I can do. Nothing I could have done."

But he'd already hung up the phone.

I sat on the bed and cried, wondering if there was anything I could have done differently. But I knew there wasn't. It was just my body. My endometriosis was rife, and it was dawning on me that I wasn't going to be able to have a baby without help. I phoned the doctor and asked for a sick note. When I picked it up, the reason it gave stated, 'recurrent miscarriage'. There it was, in black and white: my inability to carry a baby.

Simon didn't come home that weekend, but he did the weekend after. He said he'd fallen a little behind with his assignments with the drama of the miscarriage at home, so needed to stay, but I suspected he needed to stay away to have time to process what had happened. When he got home, we never talked about me losing the baby. It was like it had never happened. Maybe for him it was like that, but

I was hurting more than I had with any of the previous six. I couldn't take much more.

Simon and I coasted along until the end of November when he finished his police training and got assigned to a police station in Dingwall, a little town twenty minutes away from Inverness, so it wasn't a long commute. He was noticeably distant from me. I just thought he was still struggling to cope with our loss.

I wasn't innocent in the distance appearing between us either. I was taking extra shifts whenever they were offered to me, often working twelve-hour days. It was as though we'd lost the ability to talk to each other properly. I noticed how attached to his phone he was. He'd take it everywhere with him and when I came into our room, if he was on it, he'd quickly put it down as if he wasn't looking at it at all. I knew the signs. I wasn't stupid. But I also knew his password and, rightly or wrongly, I waited until he was sleeping one night to have a snoop and confirm or deny my suspicions. Unfortunately, my suspicions were confirmed as I read the text from the receptionist, Cara, at the station. They'd been sexting for a couple of months by the look of it. I got so engrossed in the texts I didn't even realise Simon sitting up in bed, looking at me.

"What the hell are you doing?" He asked.

I jumped out my skin and threw the phone on the bed.

"Simon. I ... uh ... Cara, Simon? Really? I know I shouldn't be snooping but I think you trump that with those messages, don't you? So, are you going to meet up with her after work when I'm working late one day, are you? Going to rip her clothes off?"

"What do you expect, Mhairi? I'm bored. You're always at work."

"Bored? You're only on your own for a few hours! I was alone every day when you were away at college. I was alone when I lost our baby. Our baby, Simon! Where were you then?"

"I didn't know what to say. I don't even know what to say now."

"Well, you know where the bloody door is if you want Cara, Simon. I won't stop you. I'm tired of feeling guilty over something I had no control over. And you weren't there for me. If this is your solution, feel free to take it."

I went to sleep that night wondering if he'd still be there the next day, or the day after that. He was, and he became less and less attached to his phone over the days that followed, until he was leaving it in the open like he used to. But I'd lost my trust in him. I felt that I needed to start putting my emotional walls up again – for self-preservation.

It took a week before Simon apologised for the sexting, and we started talking properly again.

"So, when are you thinking of starting those new tablets for your ovaries?"

"I haven't thought about it, to be honest. It's a bit scary. I don't know if I can face losing another baby. Do you really want me to try them?"

"Yeah, it couldn't hurt, could it? And if it gives us a shot of having a baby then it's worth it, I'd say. I'm settled at the station now, you're feeling better, so let's do it."

I started taking the clomiphene tablets in the second week of December. I had occasional twinges of pain, but nothing too serious, and I got right through to December 30 without anything too problematic happening. But, on Hogmanay, I woke up with excruciating cramps and obvious bloating in my womb. I was doubling over in pain when I tried to stand up. The doctors were shut, so the only thing I could do was phone NHS 24. I was put on hold while the agent contacted the hospital. When the agent came back on the phone, she told me to go into the hospital straight away. Simon drove me to the hospital where I was given a bed on the gynaecological ward. I sat on the bed and waited to be seen by one of the nurses.

"Do you know why you haven't been in sooner?" The nurse asked me when I got to the ward. "Were you not phoned on day ten of you taking your clomiphene tablets?"

"No, nobody's phoned me. Why was I meant to be seen?" I asked.

"When you take clomiphene there's a risk that your ovaries will go into hyperstimulation. You're on day twenty-one of your tablets now and I think that's exactly what has happened. I'll need to scan you inside and out to see what's going on with your ovaries."

"Oh lovely. I guess that means you'll be getting your big white wand out?" I couldn't help but giggle, but it was a nervous giggle. I felt petrified inside though. The nurse smiled at me.

"At least you still have a sense of humour. Come on, I'll take you down just now."

I got off the bed and followed the nurse down a short corridor to the ultrasound room and lay on the bed.

They took me for an ultrasound scan and a trans-vaginal scan. I lay on the bed whilst the nurse scanned first inside then outside my womb. I watched the screen as she hovered over my right ovary. Every bit of pressure she applied was painful. I tensed up and winced. The nurse turned to me.

"I'm sorry you're so sore, Mhairi," she said. "I had to press a little bit to see what was going on with your right ovary. As I thought, the clomiphene has caused hyperstimulation, but I can also see a cyst on your right ovary which will be the cause of a lot of your pain. Looks like it's about 3cm in diameter."

"What does that mean?" I asked.

"You need to stop taking the clomiphene immediately. It's obviously too much for your body to cope with, with you having endometriosis. I'm going to give you a prescription for tramadol and extra co-codamol for your pain. I'm also going to make an urgent referral back to the gynae consultant. Hopefully they'll see you within two weeks."

I cleaned myself up and Simon drove me home. It wasn't the best of ways to see in 2009.

CHAPTER 21

It was a rainy April morning when I arrived at the hospital in Inverness for the consultation for my second laparoscopy. The abdominal pains I'd had since taking the clomiphene tablets had never really gone away, even with the tramadol and co-codamol I was taking. At my appointment with the consultant, he discussed how the chocolate cyst which he'd drained in the first operation had refilled and he would need to drain it again. Chocolate cysts are common in endometriosis sufferers. The cysts fill up with brown endometrial fluid and can cause severe pain, fertility issues and often need surgical intervention,

"Can't you just take it all out now? I'm so done with the pain. Both the physical pain and the mental pain of repeatedly losing my babies. I don't know how much more of this I can take. Just take it all out. I don't care any more," I pleaded with the consultant.

"I can't do that," he said. 'You're only twenty-five. That's very young. You're still of childbearing age and you can get pregnant. And you might regret your decision later. I'm planning to remove your right ovary and fallopian tube, which will stop this cyst coming back and relieve a lot of the pain. So, you will still have one working ovary. It doesn't release as many eggs as your right one does but there's been no evidence of any cystic activity, so you have a chance of being able to conceive."

"I don't want a chance. I've really had enough. I can't take any more. Please, I am begging you. Just take everything out. I can adopt. I just want the pain to go away."

"I'm sorry, Mhairi, but taking away the right ovary and fallopian tube is really all I can do, unless I find there is something medically wrong with your left side once I'm in there. I will check, but you're just too young to make that sort of decision. You might regret your decision as you get older and more mature, and I can't just put it back. The kind of operation you are asking me to do is irreversible and life-changing".

"Fine," I replied, but I swiftly added you patronising dick in my head. I couldn't risk being removed from the consultant's 'care', so I left tearfully and waited for my surgery date.

In July 2009 I went into hospital early in the morning to have surgery to remove my right ovary and its chocolate cyst, and my right fallopian tube. The same consultant whom I'd seen in April was going to be operating on me, and he came to see me before I went to theatre in a blatant attempt to deter me from having the operation altogether.

"Now I know we've discussed this, but are you sure you want to go through with it? You will still be able to conceive, but on looking into things further, it will be far harder to do so given the infrequent ovulation from your left ovary. It will further decrease your chances of having a child," he said.

"I'm aware of this," I said. "I may be twenty-five but believe me when I tell you I'm no stranger to adversity. I know my body and the only thing you're giving me here by denying my request for a full hysterectomy is more heartache. I know you think you're doing your best, but you're far from overachieving in this instance. I'll take the ovary and fallopian tube removal but guaranteed I'll be seeing the gynae team again soon. I know the risks. Just give me the consent form and we'll be set to go."

He looked shocked, unaccustomed to such bluntness from typically worried and fragile patients. I hadn't forgotten his I know best attitude, and I was just reminding him of that. I wasn't scared as I got wheeled down to theatre, and when I woke up three hours later in the recovery room, I just wanted to be back at home. The doctor paid me another visit to let me know how things had gone.

"Your operation was as successful as it could be," he said. "I removed your right ovary and right fallopian tube as discussed and removed some endometriosis on your pouch of Douglas and sacral ligaments. The ovary and tube were stuck, both to each other and to your pelvic wall, which was a little tricky, but I managed it. I did note endometriosis on your lower left ovary which was completely stuck to your pelvic wall. I couldn't remove all the endometriosis on your pouch of Douglas so had to leave quite a bit there."

"But my left ovary isn't really going to work is it – or did you take it out because it had endometriosis on it as well?"

"No, I didn't remove it. There is still a chance that you may conceive naturally although I cannot tell you the chances of carrying full-term …"

"Still a chance that I may? So you've left me on a wing and a prayer that I might conceive and, judging by my previous seven pregnancies, miscarry again? I think we're done here. Thank you for doing the best that you can, but I don't think I will see you again." I turned my head away. I couldn't turn my body; the post-surgical pain relief was beginning to wear off, and I didn't need him to see me as weaker than I was at that point.

***

In September 2009, I received a letter from Aberdeen citing a diagnosis of 'secondary subfertility, recurrent miscarriage, severe endometriosis, persistent severe right iliac fossa pain'. Not only that, but it was also from the IVF clinic informing me I had been placed on the waiting list for an initial consultation, which I didn't even know I'd been referred for. Apparently, the consultant who had performed my operation had done it. When I looked through my medical notes, while writing this book, the consultant had written 'I will be referring her for IVF', on the day of my operation – something we hadn't discussed on that day. I was a little shocked to say the least, and I didn't feel ready to tackle IVF so soon after the last miscarriage and second operation. I needed a break from it all.

By this time, Simon was settled in his role as a constable at his police station in Dingwall. He worked long hours and did a lot of overtime. I did too at the bookmaker's, and, after countless trips to Edinburgh and Glasgow for various training courses, I soon progressed into a deputy management role. Over the winter of 2009 I filled in for the city centre shops, covering holidays and absences whilst Simon commuted the short trip to his station. But that winter was dire – they called it 'The Big Freeze' – so his twenty-minute trips could take well over an hour. My manager let me know they were opening a new shop in Dingwall in April, and I had first refusal on the deputy manager role. For me, it was an easy decision. Simon worked there, and now I could work there too. We'd talked of getting our own place and this seemed the perfect opportunity to cover all bases at once. We set our sights on a compact, three-bedroom semi, just a minute's walk from the centre of the town. It was perfect and we moved in in April, which coincided perfectly with the new shop opening.

Within a couple of weeks of moving in, I started to feel odd. I was getting twitches in my womb, and my breasts were tender and swollen. I was sick most afternoons for a couple of weeks before I realised that I could be pregnant again. Two tests confirmed my suspicions. I didn't know how to feel this time. I dared myself to be happy, but the most I could muster was flat. I went to the doctor on May 20, 2010, and he said he'd send me for an urgent early scan given my history of miscarriages and endometriosis which I was extremely grateful for. They did mention how difficult it would be to see very much at this early stage but would refer me, nonetheless. I did get a little slip of paper home with me which told me that my baby was due on January 12, 2011. I was so proud carrying that little slip of hope home in my handbag. I showed it to Simon when he got home later that day, and we just hugged each other for what seemed like ages.

"I can't believe it," he said. "This could really be it this time. Maybe that operation did the trick. It just took a little while for your body to recover."

"I hope you're right. I want to believe it so much. Until I see that scan, until I see our baby in there all safe and cosy, I can't get all hyped up yet."

I waited patiently for my scan appointment to come through whilst my baby grew inside me, wishing every day that this wee one would be the one that made it, but I never got to the appointment; never got to take the scan photo home with me. It was a warm sunny day at the beginning of June 2010 when I lost my precious baby number eight. As I sat on the bathroom floor looking through tear-filled eyes down the toilet at my dead baby, I felt any hope I had built up of being a mother disappear completely. It was over for me. Sitting on the bloody tiles, my body was broken, and my mind was overwhelmed with grief. I couldn't do it anymore. I felt so alone. My mum and dad were in Inverness and Simon hadn't come home despite the calls I'd made to his phone.

That's when I realised that I had to look after myself again. I knew Simon wanted a baby, but it was clear I couldn't give him one. I knew he loved his job, but it meant he wasn't there for me. And that day, of all the days, I needed him more than ever and he wasn't there. And that was enough for me to decide to put myself first. I had to heal my body, and I had to make my mind strong again.

CHAPTER 22

A couple of weeks later, I told Simon it was over, and I wanted out. He picked up his keys and left for about an hour, then came back.

"I've still got rights to your mum and dad's house. I want my cut if you want to split up." I had to hand it to him, he wasn't wrong. The money from Dad's clinical negligence case was nowhere near materialising at that point. I couldn't buy him out and he knew it. The only thing we could do was sell Mum and Dad's house, pay back the bank, buy him off, and leave my mum and disabled dad homeless.

I felt sick to my core. Not sick in that I wanted to physically be sick, but a deep wave of nausea that left both hatred and determination in its wake. How could he do this? It was sly and underhand, but it was also his one and only trump card. I just didn't think he would ever play it. He knew the implications his words would have if I went through with what I wanted to happen, and I hated him for it. He had stooped to the lowest of the low and now I was stuck.

"You absolute fucker! Fine. We'll play happily married for all I care. I do not want mention of babies or anything to do with them though. That's well and truly over."

So we did exactly that. I applied to become manager of my shop, as the position had recently come open. I was alone a lot of the time, while he took all the overtime he could. I spent more and more time at my parents' house when I wasn't working, and when I wasn't at their house, I was either drinking alone or out drinking with whoever was going out that night. We kept up the marriage pretence where we had to; we went to his work functions, visited his parents, who lived two-and-a-half hours away, and had holidays abroad. On the face of it, we were like any other working married couple, but I hated him.

It was at this time, in early 2011, when I should have been a mother, that my endometriosis started taking hold of me badly. Every month, I'd find myself doubled over with painful cramps, often with no warning cramps beforehand. I was changing the bed one morning, singing along to the radio. One minute, I was taking the duvet cover off. The next, I was on the floor in the foetal position, with searing pain radiating from my womb through my whole body. Pain was swiftly accompanied by the familiar multi-coloured flashing clouds in my vision, pins and needles and heat rising from my toes to my head. Then came the vomiting and diarrhoea, accompanied by huge blood clots from my womb to top it all off. I sat on the toilet for over half an hour, basin on my lap, waiting for the floodgates to shut again. It was physically and mentally exhausting, but I was in too much pain to rest properly.

I was struggling at work too. The physical toll that endometriosis took on me was huge. I was constantly tired and had no energy. The twelve-hour shifts, especially when I was on my period, were unbearable. I had to wear night pads during the day, along with super-heavy flow tampons, and I always carried spare underwear and trousers with me. I'd need to change my tampon and pad every couple of hours, but sometimes I didn't make it, and I could feel the blood running down my legs. There were times when I was serving customers with visible blood stains on my trousers – thank goodness the counters were high, but I still couldn't just walk away from customers for a quick change. I couldn't sit down either because the seats were cobalt blue fabric and I'd be risking the embarrassment of having to explain a stained chair.

My workplace then wasn't exactly accommodating to illnesses that 'weren't really illnesses' and more 'women's problems'. I remember one shift in October 2011, when I was on from 9am to 10pm. I had already been on the toilet multiple times before I got to work and, as usual, I had supplies and spares in my bags. I was also taking my full doses of co-codamol and ibuprofen religiously every four hours. The morning was quiet, so I was able to mainly concentrate on keeping my pain levels bearable – I even had my mini hot water bottle under my top. By early afternoon, I was in severe pain. I was due my painkillers again so just assumed the last lot had lost their effect. So, I took my next lot. Half an hour went by, and the pain was only getting worse. I started to double over, it hurt so much. The colleague I was working with was new and inexperienced; she couldn't manage the shop and wouldn't be able to close it at night, so I just tried my best to keep going. Eventually, the familiar-coloured dots started to appear, and my head started pounding. Sweat was pushing through my pores so quickly and furiously that I was soaking in a matter of minutes. I phoned my area manager and explained everything; just a courtesy, I thought, before going home.

"You can't just go home. There's no one to cover you. Can you not just sit there on a seat and let Kirsty do things with your supervision? Please don't turn this into a disciplinary issue," he said.

"I physically cannot work like this. I must go home. Please, I really need to go home," I said.

"You cannot go home, Mhairi. You will be in trouble and there will be consequences if you do."

Stupidly, I listened to him, and did what I was told. I did as little as humanly possible, and only helped if I absolutely had to. But I got frequently called upon, and in the end my body gave out, and I collapsed in a heap at the back of the office. I was shaking, unable to see properly and writhing in pain against the wall. At that point, Kirsty phoned the area manager to tell him what had happened, and it was only at that point that he said we could shut the shop and go home.

For me, it was too late to go home. I needed to go to the hospital. I phoned Simon to come and help me. He'd become somewhat apathetic to my endometriosis, but thankfully he did come to take me to the out of hours clinic that night. The nurse classed my collapse as an unfortunate flare-up of my endometriosis, sent me home with tramadol and told me to phone the doctor in the morning. Simon took me home, then he went back to work. That was the worst flare up of endometriosis I experienced, and it scared me a lot. I phoned the doctor the next morning and got signed off sick from work, not only for my endometriosis, but also stress, and because they started me on a treatment of Zoladex implants. These were implants that were to be injected straight into my abdomen every 28 days. Over the course of the 28 days, they would dissolve into my body, and I'd need another one. They were often used in treatment for prostate cancer in men and breast cancer in women, but also helped with endometriosis, primarily because they put you into a state of temporary menopause, meaning you didn't menstruate every month.

So, there I was, at twenty-seven, about to enter the menopause. Even though I was still married on paper, I felt so alone.

It was late 2010 when this six-foot-tall man, some years older than me, came into my shop. What first struck me was his stylish, short, silver hair, which framed his forehead, and was cut perfectly to show off his square jawline. A jawline for days, I think is what they say now. He had an air of confidence, a certain way about him. He was wearing loose, dark-grey trousers, which had flashes of fuchsia down the sides; some dark, hi-top sneakers; and a dark-grey, fitted jacket. When he came to the counter, I noticed his piercing blue eyes staring right at me.

"Hi, I'm Gary," he said. "I'm the manager of the bookies at the end of the street. Nice to meet you."

"Hi," I said. "I'm Mhairi, the manager. Looks like we're rivals."

Gary put his bet on, then he left.

We saw each other most days, nipping in and out of each other's shop to check out the customer numbers and have a general nose at our competitor's goings-on. Inevitably, we got talking a little more as time went by and started to have longer and longer conversations over the passing months. We started to confide in each other and, little by little, we realised we were in much the same position with our home lives. He'd been confined to a small attic room in his marital home, unable to split completely from his wife due to financial constraints and the fear of losing his kids. I told him of my financial predicament which bound me to Simon. We were both utterly miserable and bound in such a way that we saw no way out of our situations.

It was a horrible time for both of us but, for me, just being with him and being able to share things with him made life at home a little less awful. It didn't matter that there was eighteen years between us. We realised we were in love with each other before we were able to make the final leap away from our weird domestic set-ups. One cold winter's night we were on a works night out together. We were still 'rivals' at this point, working in separate bookies but the two shops had nights out together and got on well. Gary and I went outside for a cigarette. We looked at each other for a few seconds and then Gary wrapped his arms around me, and we kissed for the first time. It was soft and tender but passionate.

"I love you, Mhairi. I can't wait to build a life with you," he said when he pulled away.

"I love you too, Gary. I want to be with you, but I need to sort things out with the finances and the house first. I just can't risk my parents losing their house just because Simon's being a prick. As soon as my mum and dad have their house back, we can be together." I admit this, not because I'm afraid of 'being found out', but because our marriages were finished. We were living in our houses, with our legal spouses, for the purpose of having a roof over our head. There were no warm feelings, no happy memories being created, no hope of reconciliation. We were both stuck in limbo.

Gary had three kids and had been in his relationship far longer than I had been in mine. Eventually though, his financial constraints became insignificant compared to his happiness. One day whilst we were having lunch together, he told me of the latest developments at home.

"I'm moving out this week. The house is getting sold, and I am moving into my own place. I'm finally free and we can be together properly at last," he said.

"Oh my god! That's great news," I said. I was shocked that Gary had made the jump first. "I still can't do anything yet, though."

"I know, but I'll wait for you," he said.

By this time, it was Easter 2012. One morning, a couple of days after Gary told me he was moving to a new house, my mum phoned.

"Mhairi! It's all settled. The solicitor is just off the telephone. The health board has finally settled Dad's medical negligence case in full."

"Mum, that's amazing," I said. "What happens now?"

"The solicitor will send the full report to me, but the transfer of funds has already started and should be cleared in a few days."

"I'm so pleased Mum. You and Dad will finally get your house back and we'll be able to get Dad whatever he needs now. I'm so happy it's all over, even if it did take seven years of fighting for Dad!"

The settlement of Dad's clinical negligence case finally enabled Mum and Dad to pay Simon and I back for mortgaging their house and I gladly signed my name on the paperwork to give them their house back. There was a little money left over from us repaying the bank, so I suggested to Simon that we spend it all and go to Disneyland, Florida, for three weeks. Somewhere as far from reality as possible. I wanted to see if there was anything at all left of our marriage. However, our plans had to be put on hold due to my ill health.

The Zoladex injections I'd been having for my endometriosis were making me bleed painfully and unpredictably. Even when I wasn't bleeding, I was in constant pain. I was irritable, anxious, and completely exhausted. Luckily, I hadn't gotten pregnant again, but that was more to do with a lack of sex than anything. I was just grateful that I hadn't had baby number nine to worry over. I'd been for more blood tests and re-referred to gynaecology for further investigation. I'd told the doctor I really did want to have a total hysterectomy. To me, it seemed the only solution to get rid of this constant pain. However, the female doctor I saw wasn't keen, and I was met with another decision made on my behalf.

"You're still too young to consider this," she said. "You could still get pregnant and indeed you may want to in the future."

"I'm past that now. Of course, I want to, but it's pretty obvious that, although I can clearly get pregnant, I can't carry a baby to the end of the first trimester, never mind making it to term. I cannot go through that again. Not mentally, not physically. I'm telling you: I am done with the idea. My health is more important. Can you not hear me, any of you? I do not want any more pregnancies, ever. I just want it all out so I can live my life."

"I'm sorry, we just simply won't do this in someone as young as you. Tell you what; I will discuss things with another doctor, and we will decide the best course of action from here. It's not just as straightforward as 'having a hysterectomy', you know. How does that sound?"

"It sounds very much like you and another doctor are going to decide my future rather than me. Whatever you need to do to square it with yourself is fine, but I need this operation, or my quality of life isn't going to be great." I left the doctor's office feeling angry and let down.

At the same time, Dad was gravely ill. He'd been unusually quiet for a few days in early March 2012; not his usual self. Then, one morning when he got up, he was the colour of an Oompa Loompa. His skin was bright orange, and his eyes were a dirty yellow. He was more confused than usual, and he wasn't eating or drinking properly. It was scary. I couldn't ask him if he was in pain because he couldn't feel pain. Ever since his brain haemorrhage in 2005 and the damage to his nervous system that it had caused, he no longer had the ability to feel pain in large parts of his body. I spoke to Dad's doctor who got him admitted to hospital. Dad had blood tests done and had scans of his brain and abdomen. When the results came back, Dad's consultant came to talk to Mum and me.

"Allan is not a well man, as I'm sure you can see," he said. "We think he has pancreatic cancer and by the colour of him, we need to operate quickly. I can only see one way forward with this and that is to perform an operation called the Whipple's procedure. That will involve opening him up in the abdomen and taking away part of his stomach and intestine, removing the gall bladder and a section of the bile duct, then joining up what's left. It's a big operation and there is a chance, with his current medical history, that he won't make it through. But it can be successful, and the chances are he'll make a good recovery."

My mum and I looked at each other.

"What do you mean? He's not got pancreatic cancer, surely? He's been fine up until he woke up this colour," Mum replied.

"I'm afraid so," the doctor went on. "We'll have to be careful because of his shunt in his stomach though."

"There's no way he's got pancreatic cancer that bad, this quickly. We would have seen some signs of it, however small. Are you one hundred per cent sure you have this right?" I said.

"The scan shows definite shadows on the pancreas," he said.

"Could it be anything else at all? Because this operation could easily kill a healthier man, and as you said, there's his shunt in his abdomen too," I said. "He doesn't feel pain, you know. Since his haemorrhage, he wouldn't be able to tell you if he had a headache or a stomach ache. It's been us that's had to figure it out. So, pain level shouldn't be something you discount just because he says he doesn't feel it. Look…" I went over to Dad and tickled his right side. Nothing, not even a flinch. He just side-eyed me like I was being a naughty child. "Sorry Dad, just proving a point." I turned back to the doctor. "Be sure. Please be very sure and then double-check it because we nearly lost him once to a medical mistake. That won't happen again. So, if you need to re-scan him, please do it."

Mum and I were squeezing each other's hands, willing the consultant to believe us.

"I will re-scan him. Just because it is such a big operation," the doctor said.

That consultant should have been thanking his lucky stars on the day of Dad's scheduled Whipple's operation because it took until he was about to get ready for the operation for the results of the re-scans to come back and prove that there wasn't any pancreatic cancer at all. Dad had impacted gallstones. He should have been in excruciating pain with them, but he was as calm and still as ever, lighting the ward with his orange skin, and wondering what all the fuss was about. Instead of being taking down to theatre for a life-changing, possibly life-ending operation, he was taken to theatre to have his liver drained, and the gallstones removed. We got him home a few days later, more alert, looking more like a lemon than an Oompa Loompa, and, thankfully, with all his organs in one piece.

When Dad had recovered from his operation, it was finally time for Simon and I to go on our holiday to Florida. I needed the holiday in Disneyland more than ever, to take my mind off everything that had happened recently both with myself, and with Dad. I loved going on all the different themed rides and seeing the theme parks made up to resemble different films and characters. But it felt like I was there with a stranger instead of my husband. We argued most days over trivial things like which theme park we were going to on what days, or where we were having dinner. There was no hand holding as we walked round the parks, no public displays of affection like the odd cuddle or kiss, and although Simon did try to initiate sex on one occasion in the three weeks, which I refused, there was absolutely no desire to be intimate at all. It was evident that I was completely detached from Simon, and I welcomed the return home.

When I checked the mail on our return, all the final paperwork had come through to confirm Simon and I were no longer on the deeds of Mum and Dad's house. I only left it a couple of days before I finally ended things for good. Simon and I were both off work and were sitting in the living room having breakfast. I was looking out the window at the dark grey clouds which were threatening rain. I turned to Simon.

"Simon," I said. "We are done. You need to leave."

"Excuse me? I'm not leaving," he said. "This is my house too. You think this is going to be easy?"

"A lot easier than it was two years ago, yes. You have nothing to bribe me with any more. So, get out or go in the spare room, I don't care. But you will leave eventually. I've bided my time and made sure my mum and dad are safe. Now it's done and we are over. By staying, you're only fooling yourself. And you'll look like a total fool if you try and stay with me because my love for you vanished the day you threatened to make my mum and dad homeless. Now there's no possibility of that happening because our names are off the title deeds of their house."

"That was my parents who suggested that. I only said it because I was hurting. Please, I thought we were doing okay."

"Don't you think I know who suggested it? You're not clever enough to think of that yourself. You're certainly not very clever either if you think we were remotely okay after that. Your choice what you do, but either way, we are done."

For a few weeks he stayed in the spare room, until he found a house to rent just outside of town. He ran true to form when he took his belongings too. He took half of everything. I suppose this was fair enough – we were married, ergo half was his and half was mine. But when I say half of everything, I didn't expect a petty, literal division of everything. I stood in the kitchen doorway as he took an empty box into the kitchen and opened the cutlery drawer, took everything out and started separating the knives, forks, spoons and chopping knives into little piles. Then he began counting the items in each pile and separating each pile into two.

"Em, what are you doing?" I asked.

"I'm doing exactly what I am entitled to do," he said. "I'm taking what's mine and that means half of everything in this house is mine. Half of this cutlery is mine. Half the mugs. Half the tea towels."

"You are kidding me. Are you going to go through the whole house doing this? Emptying everything and separating everything so you get half of everything." I couldn't help but laugh when I spoke to him, but I saw he was serious.

"That's exactly what I'm going to do."

"You sad fuck. What about the bedroom suite and the sofas?"

"I'll only take half of them. Then you can't accuse me of taking more than I'm due."

"Oh, just take them all for goodness' sake. What possible use do I have for one bedside cabinet and whatever else you don't want?"

"I don't know but you can't stop me, unless you want to give us a chance and stay together."

"Seriously? Take your half and get out, Simon. You're pathetic. Leave your keys when you go."

I went out on the day he had hired a van to take all his stuff to his new house. He was true to his word. He took half the cutlery canteen, tealights, crockery set, numbered recipe books – all counted, separated, and split into two. A full bedroom suite – split into two – I got the dressing table; he took the bed.

When he was gone, though, I felt relieved. I slept on the sofa that was left in the living room and watched the TV, which now sat on the floor where the television unit used to be. It was just me and my cocker spaniel, Breagha.

CHAPTER 23

I coasted along in my half-furnished house for a couple of months on my own. I'd started working with Gary in his shop, so I had that to keep me occupied, and yet again I'd been back to the gynaecologist.

"Why don't we put you on the coil to help your periods," she said.

"Why don't you read my notes," I said. "That was suggested to me years ago and I refused it. I'm pretty sure that will not help me in any form. Yes, it might stop me getting pregnant, but will it stop the endometriosis?"

"It might help."

"I'm sorry, I'm past the stage of 'it might help'. I need actual help here."

"Yes, well your latest scan shows endometriosis deposits on your left ovary but it's reassuring that it is only a small amount. I'll talk to another doctor and see what they say."

"At what stage do I actually get listened to? A GP told me they'd speak to another doctor. I'm still waiting for their conversation to end apparently. It might be reassuring to you that it's a small amount given you'll never have any of this to deal with, but to me, this is affecting me every day."

"It's the best I can do."

"No. No, it's not actually."

I got up and walked out. I felt helpless. Nobody listened, nobody seemed to care.

Nobody but Gary, that is. He saw the frustration in me, and I saw how helpless he felt that he couldn't do anything about it. Unlike Simon, he was so caring and attentive. If I went into work sick, he'd make sure I had an easy shift and make me cups of tea. He just wanted to look after me.

"Why don't you move in with me now? Rent yours out and we can go halves at mine. Who cares if anyone thinks we're crazy? We've both had shite marriages and it's time we enjoyed ourselves," he said one day.

"Okay, I will. You're right, you only get one go round the board, and I couldn't care less what people think of us. We'll show them we are more than just some quick romance."

"We don't need to show anybody anything. We know we're serious, so sod everyone else."

He was right, we didn't need to. But we'd heard the whispers about us and our eighteen-year age gap; we'd seen the stares as we walked down the street. But people don't know what's on the inside, do they? People only see the surface. So I packed my house up and rented it out to a friend of a friend for enough to cover the mortgage. Gary's house was a huge, five-bedroom bungalow that his wife's friend had rented to him at a discounted price. I didn't like the idea of that at all, but we weren't in a position to be picky.

When I arrived at Gary's, it suddenly hit me that I wasn't just with him, I was with his three kids too. At that time, they were seventeen, fourteen and eleven, and had their daddy doing what they wanted, when they wanted. If something didn't go their way, they were straight on their smartphones to their mum, who would then make Gary do exactly what they wanted him to. I felt like I'd walked into a zoo at feeding time, and I was the meal. They all weren't there all the time, but when they were, it was chaos. The eldest had the biggest bedroom in the house, complete with ensuite, whilst Gary was in a room which barely held his double bed.

I admit I did not have the faintest idea of what I was doing or how to navigate it. I felt like I was back in boarding school. Although Gary and I were solid, the kids' situation was not. Our age gap didn't go down well with the kids or their mum, neither did the fact I'd moved in. Just the fact that Gary had anyone at all so quickly was a problem. There were a few nice times, of course, and when those girls laughed it would brighten up even the darkest room. They were infectious by nature and mischievously cheeky like their dad. But broken marriages create clashing sides and the old cliché 'there's two sides to every story' was made increasingly one-sided as Gary's ex-wife made sure her version of events was circulated among their old friend group, much to our detriment, of course. I couldn't take the constant undercurrent of bad feeling and I freely admit I was massively out of my depth.

In my eyes, if their own dad couldn't pacify them and explain things, then what chance did I have? So I ran away. I packed my stuff, not two months after I got there and ran back to my husband, vowing never to go back to Gary. I don't know what I was thinking. Clearly, I wasn't thinking. And as soon as I did it, I never regretted anything so much in all my life. It was clear from the minute I got back to Simon that he was gloating.

"I'll take you back, Mhairi, but I want an apology, and so do my parents. They'll forgive you in time, I suppose. Also, you need to give up work. I don't want you near Gary, or anybody else for that matter. Not for the time being."

"Okay. Fine. I'll do it. I'm just glad to be away from all that drama."

But I didn't mean it. Deep down, I was kicking myself for my rashness and stupidity. Why hadn't I gone to my parents' house and just slowed things down for a while? That would have been the obvious answer.

All I wanted was to be accepted, it was all I'd ever wanted since I was first sent away by my parents to boarding school. Bad things happen when you're not accepted, so my best option was to run. But it hurt. Even though I'd ran, I knew I had developed a love for Gary's kids that they'd never know existed, and I'd ruined the chance of showing them. After losing eight of my own babies, suddenly having three of somebody else's messed my head up. I wanted so badly to be in their lives – I never imagined that there would be forces working against us. Of course, the kids didn't know my history, my problems, or anything that would trigger me, nor should they have. I just wasn't in a good place.

After a couple of weeks, I felt like I was in a nightmare. Simon was watching my every move. Coming back from work to check on me, checking my phone and he kept asking if I'd handed in my notice at work yet. I hadn't and didn't intend to, but I couldn't tell him that until I knew what I was doing. I'd not really spoken to Gary, apart from the odd text. It was clear we were both miserable, but I wasn't sure I could ever go back to such an overwhelming situation. I remember one night Simon was driving me to my mum and dad's house, and during that twenty-minute journey, Gary called me 73 times.

"It's him, isn't it? Either block him from your phone or turn it off," Simon said.

"I can't block him, he's my boss," I replied, turning my phone off and putting it in my bag. "There, it's off. You don't have to bother about it any more. I'm not sure I want to give up work. What would I do all day? I can't just sit in the house."

"If you don't give it up then you can get out my house. You can get a hobby, look after the house. Eventually you can go back to work. I'll get a transfer somewhere and we can start again. Maybe Ullapool or somewhere further north like Thurso."

"I can't leave my mum and dad, Simon. What if something happens to Dad, and Mum needs help? She can't do it on her own. I already don't go over there enough."

"Well, that's the choice you have."

"Oh, you're fucking enjoying this, aren't you? Your little power trip? I don't think so. You aren't going to manipulate me that easily. You forget, Simon, I've been here before. Not happening again. Fine, I'll give this job up, but only when I have another one, and if you don't like it then I'll gladly leave when I can get my things out."

All this just cemented my decision that I wasn't going to be there long. He was worse than before, but the quiet way that he spoke was sneaky, and he was enjoying every minute.

"I'll let work know tomorrow that I'll have to get another job so they can start looking for a replacement. Whoever is in will tell Gary."

When I got in to work the next day, Gary was sat behind the desk, and I froze for a second in the doorway. He wasn't supposed to be in. He must have switched the rotas around so I couldn't avoid him any longer.

"Look at me, Mhairi," he said when I joined him behind the desk. "Look at me properly and tell me that you don't love me. Tell me you don't want to come back and be with me."

I turned to face him, adamant that I could do it, but as soon as I looked into his sad, glistening blue eyes, I started crying.

"I ... can't. I love you," I whispered. "I just can't deal with all the drama with your kids and your wife. It's too much."

"Come back to me. Please come back to me. I'll sort it. We will sort it ... together. Just please don't leave me alone any more without you. I need you, Mhairi. I want you. I've got nothing to offer you but me. Please just take me back. We'll be in this together. Me and you against the world."

His words hit me like the first smack of cold air hits you as you walk outside on a frosty morning. I was momentarily breathless, and, in that instant, I knew I had to go back to him.

"Okay. I'll come back. You know you're going to have a monumental shitshow to deal with though, don't you? The kids will kick off, and so will your wife."

"I don't care, Mhairi. The kids will come round in time, and she'll just have to deal with it. I mean it. It's you and me, and everybody else can either like it or lump it. We deserve to be happy."

"You best tell Sophia tonight then. I doubt that will be pretty but if you do it quick, you don't need to mull it over too long. She'll probably move out, you know. At least we can get the bigger room though, seeing as we will be paying all the bills."

"We're having it anyway. It's our home, and I don't know what I was thinking with that."

We both had a cheeky chuckle at each other.

As I expected, the next few weeks were dramatic. Simon was livid.

"I want you to give up working at the bookies and stay at home until you can prove to me and my parents I can trust you," he said.

"No way. I'm not giving up my work. You can't force me to," I replied.

"You'll do it or you can get out. Delete Gary's number, block him off everything. You can get another job when I say so."

"This was a mistake! I should never have come back to you. You want to control me now and it's not going to happen. I'm getting away from you and that's final."

I understood his anger and frustration but whether I went back to Gary or stayed at my parents I wasn't going to stay with him.

Gary's kids reacted as we'd expected them too. How could he take me back after I upset him so much? They weren't old enough or worldly wise enough to realise the complications of life – they'd led sheltered, privileged lives

– but they'd already decided they didn't want to be around us much. We just had to hope they would see things differently in time.

Eventually, Gary and I realised we just needed to be ourselves. The youngest two kids already lived with their mum, but they visited us less and less. The oldest decided to leave, unable to comprehend why her dad had taken me back. She didn't want anything to do with us. We decided it was time to downsize. The house was far too big for us to rattle around it and even with the discounted rent, the bills were too much to be comfortable with, even in 2013. We looked for weeks around Inverness and the surrounding area, but nothing suited, and we had Breagha, our cocker spaniel, with us so that added the complication of 'no pets allowed' on every rental advert.

It was only then that Mum invited us to stay at their house. It made sense. The house was big, and Mum had a lot to do on her own with looking after Dad and having the house to manage. The upstairs was pretty much unused, so it became like a little flat for me and Gary, and there were spare bedrooms, just in case any of the kids wanted to see us or stay over. I gave up working in the bookies to become employed by Dad as his personal carer. The settlement which he had received from the clinical negligence case provided funds for him to employ a full-time carer. It made sense because he'd trained me to be a carer in the nursing home where he worked, and it meant we didn't need to rely on people we didn't know coming in and out of the house. I helped Dad get washed and dressed, prepared meals, cleaned the house, took him to the toilet and made sure he was comfortable. It also meant I could give Mum a rest too and she could take some time to herself to do the things that she enjoyed, rather than having to worry about Dad all the time. Things were the calmest they had been for a long time.

CHAPTER 24

By the August of 2013, my endometriosis was the worst it had ever been before. The pain never seemed to subside, and I was on a daily cocktail of co-codamol and diclofenac. The Zoladex should have stopped my periods completely, but I was still bleeding, irregularly and very heavily. There were mornings when I'd wake up, sit on the edge of the bed for a moment and then when I stood up, I'd feel the blood come whooshing out of me and down the side of the bed and onto the carpet. In between my bouts of bleeding, I was in a menopausal state, as I was supposed to be on Zoladex, which meant I got some menopausal symptoms. Only two actually: hot flushes and night sweats. But what I lacked in the number of symptoms, I made up for with the ferocity at which I had them. Daily bed changes weren't uncommon due to the amount I sweated during the night. I'd wake up with wet pyjamas, stuck to my sweaty body, and I'd be lying in a wet patch. Gary had to stop cuddling me during the night because I was making him too hot and sweaty. I felt so guilty that my problems were now affecting him as well.

Eventually, I got seen by another gynaecologist. This time, it was an older woman. I thought, a little judgementally, that she looked of an age where she'd be experiencing some of the same symptoms, so she might be a little more supportive. I was mistaken.

"Why don't you try the pill again? Are you sure you don't want to try the coil?" she asked.

"Please don't insult my intelligence," I said. "I've been down this road before. No and no. The pill gives me migraines and neither of the two will take away this constant pain I am in with my endometriosis. Really, if there's nothing else you are going to suggest, I'm leaving and going to look into alternative options. Because not only is the Zoladex not stopping me bleeding, but I'm now menopausal whilst not being menopausal, and I have the sweats, flushes, and countless piles of washing to prove it."

"Are you not on Hormone Replacement Therapy?"

"No I'm not on HRT. Should I be?"

"Yes, you should be on it. I'll write to your GP to get that started right away. Stay on the Zoladex for now, start the HRT, and I'll see you back here in a month or two," she said.

"Thank you. I'd appreciate that." I left the appointment with a little bit of hope creeping into my head that finally somebody was trying to help me.

***

My divorce from Simon came through on my thirtieth birthday, and Gary's divorce was almost finalised too. But these milestones were overshadowed by my ongoing ill health. Three months went by, and I had heard nothing about my promised HRT. It wasn't until the April of 2014 that I eventually heard from a doctor but, by then, I'd apparently been without HRT for so long that she wanted me to go for a bone density scan to check for early signs of osteoporosis. However, the waiting list was months long, so she couldn't be sure when I would get seen. In the meantime, I started an HRT tablet, but I only lasted a month before I had to stop taking it. It calmed the night sweats and the hot flushes, but it made my endometriosis symptoms worse. The bleeding was heavier. The pain wouldn't go away, even with my painkillers, and I got cramps without warning, whether I was bleeding or not. The oestrogen in the tablet was feeding my endometriosis. I was exhausted, weak, and at my wits' end.

Towards the end of May 2014, I was back at the hospital again. Looking at my medical notes while I writing this, I see that I had been referred to as a 'nullipara' – which means a woman, or a female animal, who has never given birth. I was also described as 'this young woman… she seems very sure'. By this time, I was thirty and had been asking for years to have a hysterectomy so that I could have some quality of life, yet still I was being steamrollered by archaic views. I sat in the consultant's office, watching as she flicked through my notes for a few minutes. I stared at the floor then looked up to try and see what she was reading, then stared at the floor again, before she finally spoke.

"I see here that you've requested a total hysterectomy on multiple occasions. But you can get pregnant, and you really might regret your decision later. You're so young to give up on having children. Why don't you take your time and think about it?"

"Don't you think I've done nothing but think about it? I have lost eight babies," I said. "Does that not tell you that endometriosis is the winner here? I cannot put myself through another miscarriage again. I cannot see another baby flushed down the toilet. I cannot hope that the next baby will make it to twelve weeks, then the one after that might make it to fourteen or fifteen. How plain do I have to make it? And my partner has three children and has had the snip, so even if there was a remote chance I wanted to risk pushing myself over the edge, he's firing blanks."

"You might split up with him and get another partner later on …"

"I'll stop you there. Don't even go down that road. I've had enough. It's my body. Either you're going to listen to me or you're not. Which one?"

"You'll need HRT until you're at least fifty. Which reminds me, I'll change that HRT you're on to a newer one, and we can see how you go on that. I will look at your last MRI scans from 2012 and maybe get another scan and then we will go from there."

"I'll believe it when I see it, and I'm sorry but you haven't left me with much confidence."

***

I still hadn't had my bone scan appointment. My mum and dad were appalled. I don't think they'd realised just how bad I had been with the endometriosis until I had moved back in. They were used to seeing me in pain, used to me curled up on the couch with the dogs looking colourless when Gary was at work. Mum told me she was looking up a private clinic to get my bone scan done. Within a week of her finding the number, I'd been for my scan and got my results of osteopenia – I had pre-osteoporosis. The months I'd not been on HRT whilst being on Zoladex had weakened my bones enough for the doctors to be a little worried about them. It was just another ailment in my long list to worry about. By the end of September, I had heard nothing about whether I would be able to get a hysterectomy or not, so I went back to the doctor. She had also heard nothing. Out of desperation, I asked if I could just get the ovary out, just to speed things up and I was promised a speedy reply. One month later, I still hadn't heard anything.

"That's it!" Mum yelled through from the kitchen as I was greeting the dogs. "You're going private. I can't see you going through this any more. You have a look online and do a bit of research to find someone you think you can trust and who has the experience, and your dad and I will pay for you to get whatever needs done. You can't live like this any more."

"Are you sure? It won't be cheap."

"I don't care how much it costs. We have the money there. You need a specialist to look at you and those chocolate teapots you've seen so far need a good slapping. Just tell me when you've found someone."

"Thank you so much. I mean it. I'm so grateful." I had tears falling down my cheeks. It was like a weight being taken off my shoulders.

"I just want my wee girl to be okay. You're no right and we need to get you well." Dad piped up. It wasn't something he often did, give a lucid contribution to a conversation but the fact he had showed just how much he was taking notice of how ill I had become. I wrapped my arms around him.

"Thanks Dad."

"Anything so long as you get better."

Within a couple of days, I'd found the consultant I wanted to see. He was based in Edinburgh at a Spire clinic and had a vast range of experience in gynaecology. His specialisms were specific, and endometriosis was one of them. I was convinced I'd found the right person. I phoned the clinic, and they booked me in for a consultation on November 4, 2014. When Gary and I entered the room, we were holding hands tightly. We had no idea what was in store. The room was bright and spotlessly clean and set out like a standard doctor's office but with comfortable black leather seats a real plant in the corner by the window. The consultant was unassuming but had a kind and trusting face. He wore a charcoal grey suit with a white shirt that gave him a professional, yet casual look and he had an air of confidence about him that put me at ease straight away. He had my medical notes in a pile on the desk.

"I've read through all your notes, Mhairi. Before we discuss them, I'd like to give you a quick physical examination just to check a few things and then we can have a discussion. Okay?"

I nodded and hopped up onto the bed. Five minutes of prodding and poking later, with a few 'hmms' and 'mm-hmms' thrown in, I was back sat beside Gary, holding his hand.

"It's okay. Don't look so frightened," the doctor said.

"Honestly, I'd love to be positive right now, but this has been a very long, hard road," I said.

"I can see that. Well, I have good news and bad news ..."

"Bad news first, please. I don't want to leave here feeling worse than I came in."

"Well, there's absolutely no chance of you carrying a pregnancy to term. I can feel adhesions all over the place."

"Eight miscarriages later, I can agree I won't carry a pregnancy full term."

"I know. It's horrible for you. I cannot understand why you've just been left to get on with this. In my opinion, you're the ideal candidate for a total hysterectomy. I think it would be cruel not to give you that. You're completely right to be asking for one."

I couldn't help it. I burst out crying. "You're kidding?" I managed to blubber.

"Not at all. You clearly can't go on like this and as far as I can see, this is your only and best option. I see no reason to delay this. All the evidence points to the fact that you should have a hysterectomy. The only thing I will need to do is get you in for a quick MRI scan to both give me a recent image of what's going on and where everything is, and also make sure that I can do this via keyhole surgery rather than opening you up. I need to warn you that I might need to open you up once I start the operation, if things are proving to be a bit trickier than I'd expected. There are the usual risks to having a general anaesthetic, but the nurses will go through that with you. Because of the delicate organs in the area, namely your bladder and bowel, I do need to warn you of the risk of damage to either or both of those. Worst case scenario is a colostomy bag and a catheter. How does that sound?"

I looked at Gary, his face visibly losing what little colour it had, and gave his hand a little squeeze.

"Honestly, it sounds amazing. Thank you so much. Thank you for listening to me and not just seeing my age. I'm so grateful. Will I need to book the scan at reception?"

"Actually, I'll give them a quick ring and see what their slots are. They may well squeeze you in for me."

I put my head on Gary's shoulder and he looked down at me and put his hand on my cheek. He mouthed "You okay?" I nodded and smiled.

"There's a slot later today if you are okay with that?"

"Yeah, that's fine," I replied, looking at Gary for reassurance.

"That's fine with me," he echoed.

A few minutes later, everything had been arranged. I would come back later in the day for the scan. The consultant had promised to get back to me as soon as possible with the results. I didn't expect the phone call to come at 8pm the next night though.

"Hi Mhairi. I've got your results in front of me," the consultant said. "As far as I can see, everything will be fine for me to perform the hysterectomy via keyhole. I can't foresee any problems based on the scan, and I am absolutely sure that you're making the right decision here. Given your response to the Zoladex, it's the right thing to do. The only drawback is the length of time you will be on HRT, but that doesn't seem to faze you. So if you're happy, I'll get you booked in?"

"That's great news," I said. "Yes, I'd like to get booked in. Shall I phone the clinic in the morning?"

"No, no. I've got my diary here. I'm free on December 3 if that suits you. If it does, I'll let the clinic know in the morning and then they'll send out everything you need."

Finally, I felt like I had someone on my side and there was an end to my pain-filled days in sight.

CHAPTER 25

On December 2, 2014, Gary and I left Inverness and drove the three hours down the A9 to Edinburgh. We'd booked a room at the hotel next door to the clinic, as I had to be there for seven o'clock the next morning. We'd planned a lovely day out at Edinburgh Zoo before going for a Chinese meal. I was determined to enjoy myself, mainly because I was panicking that I would die during the operation. The seriousness of what I was about to go through had crept up on me suddenly. I was thirty and about to go through a life-changing operation that, although I was certain it was the right thing to do, seemed risky. I knew the consultant wouldn't fully understand the extent of the damage the endometriosis had done until he was foraging about inside me with various cutting and prodding tools.

I could wake up and have a colostomy bag or a catheter for the rest of my life. I could have nerve damage. The possibilities just kept swirling through my head and shivering my way round Edinburgh Zoo was the perfect distraction. If you've ever been to Edinburgh Zoo, you'll know that it sits on an almighty hill that knackers even the nimblest of us. The pain I was in climbing that hill that day served only to affirm my decision about my upcoming hysterectomy.

The next morning, Gary drove me round the corner from the hotel to the clinic. A nurse took us into a private room. There was a hospital bed, locker, chair, and bed table, like you would see in any other hospital, but I also had an ensuite shower room and a TV. It was basic, but spotlessly clean, and the bed was comfy with squishy pillows and a warm duvet on it. Before long there were nurses coming in and out, filling out information on forms and double-checking I was who they thought I was. The anaesthetist came in and explained what she was going to do.

"I'll just put a needle in the back of your hand, pop a couple of syringes in and the next thing you know, you'll be back in here all cosy in bed."

"Can you not just stick a mask over my face to knock me out?" I don't know where the sudden fear of getting a needle in the back of my hand came from, but there it was. "It's going to hurt so much."

"I promise it won't. I'll be gentle and you will only feel a scratch. Tell you what, I won't put it in until we are down in my room though, okay?"

"Perfect." I looked to Gary who was trying to smile through his worry. "I don't know where that came from. All that endo-pain and I'm afraid of a needle! Stupid, I know."

"Stupid? You're the bravest person I know. You're just taking all this in your stride like it's nothing. You're coping way better than I ever would."

"I'm doing a good job of covering it up, then?"

"A perfect one," he smiled.

There was a gentle knock at the door.

"Morning, Mhairi. Hi Gary." It was my consultant, looking very energetic for 8am. "Have you been getting the Spanish Inquisition from everyone? I think we're just about ready to go. Any questions?"

I shook my head.

"Good stuff. Well, you've got a good team looking after you and I don't anticipate any problems, so we should be ready for you in the next half hour or so. I'll see you down there."

"Hopefully I won't see you, though."

He chuckled as he left the room and there was no turning back. About twenty minutes later a nurse came to take me down to theatre.

"I love you, Gar. You be here when I wake up?"

"Course I will, my wee Mhairi. I'm going to nip back to the hotel and freshen up, go and get some snacks for later and I'll be right here. Might get us a DVD to watch 'cos there's a DVD player on the telly. Love you loads."

And with that, I walked with the nurse down to the anaesthetic room attached to the theatre. I got up on the trolley, lay back and shut my eyes as I began to get hooked up to machines. I was so pre-occupied by the goings-on that I never even felt the needle going into my hand.

"All right, Mhairi. We're good to go. Just listen to my voice. I'm going to get you nice and comfy. You should feel a cold sensation in your arm. Just start counting slowly, backwards from ten for me."

"Ten ... nine ... eight ... seven ... si ... six ... fi ..."

***

"Where's Gary? Gary? I want Gary!" The room was blurry, and I was so confused.

"Mhairi? Don't worry, sweetie. You're in recovery. Everything is okay. Gary is in your room waiting for you. I'm just going to give you some painkillers, okay?" Everything went fuzzy and I shut my eyes. The next time I opened them I was in bed in my room. I could feel a dull throbbing from my waist down.

"Gary. You're there."

"I'm here, Mhairi. Don't worry. You're okay. You've had your operation. Try not to move too much. Have a rest."

The next few hours went by, dipping in and out of a morphine-induced sleep. I was aware that Gary was there, and I was conscious of nurses coming in and out, the blood pressure cuff on my left arm tightening and loosening to check there was no internal bleeding. Around teatime I woke up properly, my throat like sandpaper from the tubes that had been inserted during my operation. The pain was more acute now, focused from my belly button down to my thighs, and I was aware of a weird sensation in my bladder. I pulled the cover back and saw the catheter.

"What the hell is that? Please tell me that can come out!" I panicked.

"It's just temporary," Gary said. "Just while you get back on your feet. You might be glad of it for the next few hours."

"Absolutely not! That's coming straight out when a nurse comes in." I didn't need to wait long. About ten minutes later, a nurse came in the room.

"Hello Mhairi. Glad to see you're awake. How are you feeling?" she asked.

"Like I've been run over by a stampede of wildebeest. Other than that, perfect. Please can you take this catheter out. It's such a horrible feeling. I'll get up and go for a wee myself."

"I don't think you're quite ready for that yet. Let's just keep it in overnight and see how you go."

"Honestly, I'm ready for it. Please take it out. It's a horrible feeling. If I can't manage, I promise I'll let you know. Gar, will you help me to the loo?"

The nurse and Gary gave each other a concerned look. Gary looked round to me and nodded.

"Okay. But please do not be struggling to go for a wee," said the nurse. "You've had a big operation, and you need to be careful." She came closer and drew back the covers. I looked down and saw three little dressings dotted round my belly and pelvic bone, and the tell-tale tube draped over my leg leading to the urine bag. My belly was huge, still filled with all the gases used to inflate my insides during the hysterectomy. I felt the tube slide out of me and then the sense of relief when it finally plopped onto the bed. Gary and the nurse helped me to sit on the edge of the bed and it took me a few minutes to catch my breath. The anaesthetic hadn't fully worked its way out of my system, but I was determined that I would get up and moving. I stood up, wobbly on my feet and with Gary supporting me, made the few steps to the toilet and managed to pee. That was the first hurdle out of the way. It knackered me and I was glad to get helped into bed again.

"I bought you a DVD when I was out at the shop. The Secret Life of Walter Mitty. I'll stick it on for us. More to keep me amused, I think."

Gary was right, I can't remember anything about the film. Apparently though, I was awake for some of it.

By teatime, I was ready for some food, and managed to plough my way through dinner and pudding. Gary stayed with me until around 9pm, then went back to the hotel. I spent the night drifting in and out of short bouts of sleep. The night nurse was amazing and took care of me all night. She brought cups of tea, and sat and chatted with me, making sure I was fully dosed up on painkillers. She even brought me biscuits. I was so grateful for her going out of her way to make me so comfortable.

When Gary came back in the morning, I was feeling in need of a freshen-up. The nurses offered to help, but I only wanted Gary to help me. He was so careful with me and gentle, like he was washing a cracked porcelain cup. Afterwards, there was a knock on the door, and in came my consultant.

"Morning, guys. How are you? Oh, look at you, Mhairi. You look better. I nipped in yesterday, but you were out cold, so I decided to leave you be until today. So, the operation went well. Your uterus was tilted backwards and fixed in place with lots of endometriosis. There were lots of deposits round the pouch of Douglas. I'd rate your endometriosis as severe. Even though you've been on Zoladex for a long time, there was still a lot of active endometriosis on your womb, your cervix and in your left ovary and fallopian tube. I managed to remove most of it. However, I had to leave some on your bladder and bowel, because I really risked damaging those if I tried to cut the endometriosis away. But still, I am one hundred per cent sure that you have made the right decision here. I'm just sorry you had to fight for it for as long as you did."

"So that's it? I'm free of it?"

"For the most part, yes. You might get residual pain from time to time because of the endometriosis that's still there. But your body won't be producing oestrogen like it was before, so the endometriosis should remain inactive. The HRT shouldn't wake it up. I can't give you a cast-iron guarantee that you'll never feel pain, but you're certainly never going to have to deal with that level of suffering from endometriosis again."

"Thank you so much. I'm so grateful." I burst into tears. Years of pain ruling my life had ended because somebody finally listened to me. "Please can I go home now?"

"Yes. I'll see you in a few weeks just to make sure you're okay."

The three-hour journey back up the road to Inverness was horrible. I felt every bump in the road like I was being punched in the pelvis. Every corner was like an out-of-body experience, with my body fighting against the sway of the car. I wasn't fully awake, having been dosed up on heavy painkillers ahead of the journey, but I was aware of everything at the same time. Although Gary was driving slower and gentler than usual, it didn't stop my groans and grumbles over every bump and pothole. Eventually we arrived home, and I went straight to bed, completely wiped out. The relief of finally having the operation combined with being in my own cosy bed with the dogs by my side, and Gary and Mum flitting about helping me made it possible to finally relax.

I stayed in bed for a couple of days, only getting out to go to the toilet and wash. Then, I managed to go into our living room and wander about for short spells upstairs for a few days. Eventually I made it downstairs, which made it easier for when Gary was at work. Slowly, I could feel myself healing, along with the realisation that the endometriosis pain wasn't returning. For the first time since I had been fourteen years old when I had had my first period, I could imagine a future where I was pain free and not having to rely on painkillers to get through a day.

CHAPTER 26

In the weeks and months that followed my hysterectomy, I gradually got my strength back. Even though I'd had the operation through keyhole surgery, I still had to be careful with lifting or strenuous activity. I felt like a fraud having to rely on Gary, who was working full-time, and my mum, who was recovering from pancreatitis, to do all the washing and hoovering and walk the dogs. Every little thing that I began to be able to do again felt like a little part of me coming back, before once again I was able to do everything myself and get back to helping Mum and Dad again. After Mum had her pancreatitis scare, and I was in recovery, I think Mum and Dad started to feel isolated in Inverness. Gary and I felt the same, but we didn't mind where we lived so long as we had each other.

"I want to move," Mum said one day. "I think it would be good if we went back down to Fife. All the extended family is there." It was a shock, but it made sense.

"Dad, what do you think?" I asked him.

"Me? I'm not bothered," he said. "I just want a quiet life. But it will be the last time I move anywhere. Next time it will be in a box."

"Fair enough," I said. "We'll need to get somewhere big enough to live together though. If not together then close by because you'll need help Dad, and Mum, sorry but you're not getting any younger and if Dad falls or there's an emergency, you can't deal with that alone. Gar, what do you think?"

"I'm with your dad. I just want a quiet life. With you, Mhairi. Where you go, I go. That's all that matters to me."

"I guess that's that settled then. Let's get this on the market. Will you start looking for somewhere, Mum?"

Within a couple of weeks, our Inverness house was on the market, and Mum had found and put in an offer on a property not far from St. Andrews, Fife. It was a large house for Mum and Dad, with a workshop on the same grounds that had been converted into a two-bedroom cottage, ideal for Gary and me. The large house had originally been a farmer's cottage from the 1800s, and the original part of the house had walls that were two-feet thick. Over time, extensions had transformed the cottage into a five-bedroom, three-bathroom house that looked backed onto a forested area and had views across the Fife countryside. It was ideal for having friends and relatives to stay, and had enough space to accommodate carers later down the line when Dad might need them.

Our cottage was like a little lodge house. It had previously been a garage, then a workshop, then had been transformed into a little cottage with a galley kitchen, open-plan living room and dining room, then a steep staircase up to a little shower room and two bedrooms with sloped ceilings on either side. The garden was shared at the back, but each house had a little private area at the front door. Between the two houses was a large lawn with two decking areas overlooking an old chicken coop, wild shrubs and bramble bushes and a large wooden lodge which would be Gary's man cave where he could listen to his collection of vinyl at an insanely loud level. It was perfect for us all.

Gary's divorce had finally come through, so we decided that 2015 was going to be our year to get married. We didn't want a big do, and even if we did, Gary's kids were out of the picture. They lived with their mother and although attempts had been made to have a relationship with them, they still weren't accepting of Gary and I. My family was scattered across the UK. So we decided we would elope to

Gretna Green. It suited us perfectly. We'd both had the big white weddings and all the fanfare and expenses that go with it. This was something just for us to celebrate our love for each other.

We booked a package wedding for September 16, 2015. All we needed were our outfits, and a bouquet for me. Gary bought a navy suit for under £200, and a silk, floral scarf. I bought a long, fitted dress in pale browns and nudes, with delicately sequined flowers and sheer netting that cost £150. My bouquet was made of silk roses, complementing the dress perfectly, and it only cost £30 as an ex-display piece. I booked a lady local to the Gretna Green area to do my hair and make-up. The most expensive items were our rings. I chose mine from a high street jeweller, a white gold ring with a single diamond set in a claw. Gary got his wedding ring made from silver, with black onyx set in the top.

In homage to where we met – the bookies – we spent the day before our wedding at Carlisle racecourse. Our wedding morning was fuss-free and relaxed, as I sat and got my hair and make-up done with a coffee. We were picked up by a lady in a chauffeur's cap, driving a vintage cream Rolls Royce, which transported us to the famous blacksmith's shop, where English and Welsh lovers would elope to from the late 1700s. Blacksmiths who conducted weddings for runaway couples would strike the anvil with a hammer to signify the marriage was complete.

As we stood in front of the famous Marriage Anvil, reciting our vows in front of the registrar and two witnesses we'd never met before, we both had tears in our eyes. As I looked at Gary, I thought, This is it. All my struggles with endometriosis, all my mental turmoil, through everything since the day we met, you've been there. You've never lifted a hand to me. Never thrown anything at me. Never even threatened it. Sure, we've had some blazing, Oscar-worthy arguments, but never in my life have I felt as safe as I do with you. There has never been, nor do I think there will ever be a day when I don't feel safe with you.

After the ceremony, we had our photos taken and then were driven back to our hotel where a private room had been made up for us to enjoy our wedding meal. The whole day was perfect – Gary and me doing what we'd always done, sticking together.

When we returned home the day after our wedding, my sister had driven up from Blackpool with her boyfriend and there was a wedding cake waiting for us.

"You didn't think you'd get away with not having anything at all waiting for you, did you?" asked Mum. "We had to have some sort of celebration with you. You two deserve it after everything."

It was such a lovely surprise for us and a nice little get-together before we packed our cases and took the dogs away for our two-week honeymoon at the Ardnamurchan peninsula on the west coast of Scotland. It was our little slice of solitude before we picked up our lives to move to Fife.

For Mum, Dad, and me, the move would mean we would be returning to our roots in our home county. For Gary it turned out that he, too, was returning to his ancestral home county. Most of his paternal family going back over 150 years had been born less than five miles from our new house that we had bought. It was a new beginning for all four of us. By the time we moved we still had no contact with Gary's kids who were by now twenty, eighteen and fifteen. We didn't even know their address in Inverness, though through the grapevine we'd heard they'd moved for the third or fourth time. The oldest girl was living away from her mother and two sisters in a flat she rented. It was a sad situation, but we needed to make our own life and be happy together. We always held on to the hope that things would change at some point in the future, but we couldn't press pause on our lives to wait for something that may or may not happen. We just knew that a fresh start would do us all the world of good. And I knew that after all the abuse and trauma that I had been through in my thirty-one years of being alive I could finally be happy in my own mind and truly proud of the woman I had become.

ACKNOWLEDGEMENTS

My first thanks is to Stuart at Chiselbury Publishing who took a chance on me and my story. Without you there would be no book and I will be forever grateful.

Thank you to my editors, David Haviland and Rhodri Owen who helped make sense of the story I was trying to tell.

A huge thank you to Nancy and Marian who helped the family out when I was away on my writing breaks.

To my mum and dad, Joyce and Allan. Much of this book is about our relationship so know that I love you both always and I am here for you.

To my (step) daughter Eireann and my grandson, Wren. To me, there is no 'step'. I love you as if you were my own, and having that love in my life has allowed me to deal with my past losses. Wren, when you came along you gave me those years I missed as a mother in Eireann's life.

Last, but not least, to my darling husband, Gary. You have supported me and encouraged me from the first thought I had of putting my life down on paper, and continue to do so. Without you by my side, and without our constant video calls and texts whilst I was away reliving the traumas of my past, I could not have done this. You kept me sane and strong. I love you with all my heart.